This Book Will
Make You Sleep

Dr Jessamy Hibberd
and
Jo Usmar

Quercus Editions Ltd
55 Baker Street
7th Floor, South Block
London
W1U 8EW

First published in 2014

A CIP catalogue record for this book is available from the British Library

ISBN 978 1 84866 287 2
Printed and bound in Great Britain by Clays Ltd, St Ives Plc

10 9 8 7 6 5 4 3 2 1

Designed for Quercus Editions Ltd by Peggy Sadler at Bookworx
www.bookworx.biz

Contents

A note from the authors

We live in ever-changing times and sometimes life can be tough. We're constantly being pulled in different directions and can struggle to cope with the pressure that we're put under by external factors and, most importantly, by ourselves. With greater choice comes greater responsibility and occasionally this can be a breeding ground for stress, unhappiness and self-doubt. There are very few people (if any at all) who feel they operate perfectly in their work, relationships and life in general. Most of us could use some help now and then – a nudge to show us how to improve our mood, to change our approach to life and to feel more content.

This series aims to help you understand why you feel, think and behave the way you do – and then gives you the tools to make positive changes. We're not fans of complicated medical jargon so we've tried to make everything accessible, relevant and entertaining as we know you'll want to see improvements as soon as possible. These concise, practical guides show you how to focus your thinking, develop coping strategies and learn practical techniques to face anything and everything in more positive and helpful ways.

We believe self-help doesn't have to be confusing, worthy or patronising. We draw on our professional experience and the latest research, using anecdotes and examples which we found helpful and hope you will too. Titles are split into particular areas of concern such as sleep, happiness, confidence and stress, so you can focus on the areas you'd most like to address.

Our books are based on a Cognitive Behavioural Therapy (CBT) framework. CBT is an incredibly successful treatment for a wide variety of issues and we're convinced it will enable you to cope with whatever you're facing.

Within the books you'll regularly come across diagrams called mind maps. They are easy to use and simple to understand. Based on CBT, mind maps show how your thoughts, behaviour and how you feel (both emotionally and physically) are all connected, breaking the problem down so it doesn't seem overwhelming, and laying out options for making changes.

There are exercises and checklists throughout, to guide you through the practical steps of altering how you feel. We'll make it easy to make these changes part of your routine because reading the theory is only going to get you so far. The only way to ensure you'll feel better long-term is to put everything you learn into practice and change how you experience your day-to-day life.

You can *choose* to feel better and these books will show you how.

Good luck! Let us know how you get on by contacting us on our website: www.jessamyandjo.com.

Jessamy and Jo

Introduction

Snoozing, slumber, forty winks, shuteye – whatever you call it, sleep is an integral part of all our lives. You can't *choose* to stop needing sleep, just like you can't choose to stop breathing. It's a function that our bodies perform automatically, which means not being able to drop off can be frightening, frustrating and completely exhausting.

We spend about a third of our lives asleep on average, or at least we're supposed to if all goes according to plan. However, when you're lying in bed counting down the hours until your damn alarm goes off, the helplessness you feel can become overwhelming; it can start affecting your day-to-day life. When you're sleeping normally you don't even think about it, yet when it goes wrong sleep can become an all-encompassing obsession. It's like getting toothache – the pain is suddenly all you think about, influencing everything you do and how you feel. When you can't sleep you'll curse yourself for not appreciating those blissful nights of oblivion you used to know.

We have to sleep to survive – you're not just conked out, your body is going through extraordinary psychological and physiological processes. In fact, you can actually survive better without food than you can without sleep. The harder your body and brain works during the day the more you need to rest, which is why the consequences of sleep deprivation can be dramatic.

In spite of all this, it's harder than ever to switch off in the modern world. After a day at work we come home to TV, the internet and a flurry of Facebook notifications, Tweets and more emails (work and personal). Smartphones are starting to become the norm, bringing the Internet and social media into every aspect of our lives – constantly distracting us and making it that bit harder to wind down.

The good news is that while you can't force sleep, there are loads of things you can do to encourage it. This book aims to give you the means to kick-start positive resting patterns, whether your sleep's been messed up for a night, a week, a month or a year.

Sleep problems

This book deals with problems specifically associated with falling asleep, staying asleep, waking early and insomnia. We're not covering issues such as sleep-related breathing disorders, restless leg syndrome, sleep walking, narcolepsy, hypersomnia, night terrors or other parasomnias.

If you're suffering from any of the conditions listed above, or if you've been suffering from severe sleep issues for a long time, you should consider visiting your GP to get yourself checked out; you might need specialist help.

The techniques and strategies we recommend in this book will kick-start more natural sleeping patterns and these will work alongside your GP's treatment – so you could take a two-pronged approach.

Why is sleeplessness affecting you?

There are lots of reasons why you might not be able to sleep: stress, an important life event, a change in your sleeping environment, health issues, etc. Or perhaps you've not been getting enough rest for ages and have just accepted constant tiredness as a way of life.

Sleeplessness can be exceptionally lonely (especially if you've got a partner snoring merrily beside you). It can make you feel demoralised, demotivated and pretty angry. However, please be reassured that you're absolutely not alone. At any one time 25 per cent of the UK population and approximately 50–70 million Americans will be suffering from a form of sleep disorder that affects their daily lives. While that might not be much comfort, it should make you feel less like the only person on earth counting increasingly panicked sheep at 3a.m.

In today's fast-paced 'have it all' society there never seems to be enough hours in the day to squeeze everything in – and sleep can be the first thing to suffer. You might sacrifice hours in bed for work or socialising or lie there thinking about everything you have to do tomorrow. Unfortunately sleep isn't expendable so any negative patterns you fall into will play havoc with your body clock. When you're stressed about not sleeping you can inadvertently end up doing things that make your situation worse. The way you think gets all messed up, which makes you behave differently, leaving your body feeling run down and your emotions all over the place.

As intimidating as tackling sleeping issues can seem there are simple and effective ways of getting things back to normal and rebuilding your positive associations around going to bed.

Who we are and what this book's about

Lack of sleep will affect most people at some point in their lives – which is why we've written this book. We have both experienced the mind-numbing tedium and then the panic of lying awake at night and feel a book such as this could have helped. Everything you'll find in here is concise, accessible and hopefully relatable. The easy-to-adopt strategies and techniques that we recommend will help you both now and in the future. (We have also included a list of resources for further reading and help in the back of the book.) We hope like-minded people recognise themselves in what we've written, and that it will help them feel much more confident in managing their sleep problems.

Sleep affects how you think, behave and feel both emotionally and physically so addressing the problems will, and we're not exaggerating, change your life.

How the book works

This is a really practical book – a manual to sleeping better. We strongly advise that if you want to make long-term positive changes you invest time in the strategies. The techniques we recommend are proven to work. You need to break your bad sleeping habits and make positive new ones.

While some activities will have an immediate impact, others may take time and practice in order to become second nature. It's like anything – the more you work at it the easier it becomes. If you adopt these techniques into your day-to-day life we're 100 per cent convinced your sleeping patterns will improve.

We'll show you how to use a sleeping diary to help you understand how you sleep (see Chapter 3). It may sound like a drag, but it is brilliantly effective. Writing things down makes you think logically and rationally (two of the first thought processes to fly out of the window when you're exhausted) about what's actually going on and how you really think and feel about sleep. It's is a great way to break down problems, making them more manageable, and it'll provide inspiration when you look back and see how far you've come.

As previously mentioned we have used a Cognitive Behavioural Therapy framework (see Chapter 2) throughout the book as it's a highly effective, problem-focused approach that deals with the here and now. You'll learn a set of principles which will help you to deal with your sleeping problems and that will stay with you for the rest of your life.

How to get the most out of the book

+ Read the chapters in order as each one builds on the last.
+ Invest time in all the strategies (identified by the symbol **S**) rather than just blitzing through some and ignoring others. These techniques work! By trying them all you'll be giving yourself the best possible shot at sleeping better.
+ Buy a new notebook and dedicate it to this book. Several of our strategies involve writing things down or drawing them out (including the diary already mentioned). Writing things down will make them 'official' and seeing how far you've come will be very motivational.
+ Breaking bad habits can take a while (approximately twenty-one days) so please don't get despondent if you're not sleeping like a

baby immediately. The strategies will work for you if you stick with them.

Sleeplessness is not something you have to accept. You *can* wrestle back control and start looking forward to going to bed again.

I

While You Were Sleeping

This chapter explains what sleep actually is, why we need it and what kind of things can scare it off. Understanding why you're tossing and turning will help to pinpoint the things you need to focus on to sleep better.

What is sleep?

Sleep is a curious beast and trying to discover exactly what happens when we drop off has provoked many a restless night for scientists. The processes we go through when snoozing are extraordinarily complex, however there is one thing that everyone agrees on: sleep is essential to maintaining a functioning brain and body. Without it we'd turn into zombies (a state you might recognise after pulling an all-nighter).

Sleep gives us a chance to recover and regenerate. It's an active process – while you're dreaming of winning the lottery and skipping through fountains of champagne, your body is undertaking activities vital for life. Sleep affects our ability to use language, sustain attention and summarise what we see and hear. Our brains busily filter information, making memories and picking out emotional details to create new insights and ideas. What we've learned during the day gets organised, setting in motion how we feel and act when we wake up. And that's just the psychological side – the physical processes are dramatic too. Your body is relaxed into a state of paralysis to stop you acting on your dreams and the endocrine system (the collection of glands that regulate such things as metabolism, growth and repair) kicks in, secreting hormones that keep you asleep.

Sleep: the facts

Sleeplessness is one of the most common complaints heard by doctors. 51.3 per cent of adults in the UK struggle to drop off at night with one in ten suffering from insomnia (a persistent inability to obtain adequate uninterrupted sleep). This alarming stat jumps to one in five in people over sixty-five years old. It's perhaps unsurprising then that sleeplessness is considered a major public health problem. The Office for National Statistics conducted a large study investigating the most common health concerns amongst the UK's general population in 2001 and sleep disturbance and fatigue were by far the most frequently reported worries. Those sufferers also reported how insomnia dramatically affected their mental and emotional health.

This isn't just a UK problem by any stretch of the imagination. The equivalent of billions of pounds is spent worldwide every year on prescribed medications, over the counter remedies and other sleep solutions. The US Behavioral Risk Factor Surveillance System Survey (2009) found that 37.9 per cent of the 74,571 American people surveyed reported unintentionally falling asleep during the day at least once in the preceding month. This isn't only inconvenient (and potentially embarrassing), it could also be very dangerous.

Sleep is something you have to do. You're programmed to do it and can't stop your need for it no matter how hard you might try. All of which means it's pretty hideous if sleep remains elusive even when you're totally exhausted. Don't panic though. This book will help you to cope with and quickly overcome problems associated with both sleep deprivation and disturbance.

Levels of sleep deprivation

Everyone is different and so the quality and amount of sleep people need varies hugely. Contrary to popular belief, there is no generic 'perfect' number of hours to suit everyone. Most adults, on average, sleep for between seven and eight and a half hours per night. However, some people will be able to function perfectly well on as little as four hours (only about 1 per cent of people are this lucky according to Loughborough University's sleep centre) while other people may need nine or ten. There is no general consensus or golden rule. Sleep is completely and utterly individual. You may need six hours a night to be at your best while someone your exact same gender, age, height and weight needs eight. How your body balances the amount of sleep it needs with the amount of sleep it's getting can't be summarised or guessed at. This is why you have to trust how you actually feel – physically and mentally – rather than how you think you should feel. If you feel exhausted after only getting five hours a night that's a pretty good indication that you need more than five hours a night. Your body won't lie to you.

How a lack of sleep will affect you is also completely personal. Experiments in sleep deprivation are seldom undertaken due to the ethical concerns surrounding such practices. Some tests conducted in the 1950s and 1960s (which raised a lot of eyebrows over the risks involved) illustrated just how important sleep is. The physical and emotional effects on the test subjects after prolonged sleep deprivation were dramatic – which is why not allowing someone to sleep is a particularly vicious form of torture. We have to sleep to survive.

Your age, lifestyle, diet and how you think about sleep all play a part in influencing the amount of time you need to spend in bed. Changing how you think and feel about slumber is a key part of being able to sleep better – whether you have occasional bad nights, regular sleepless weeks or you suffer from insomnia.

What is insomnia?

Insomnia is a persistent problem with sleep for at least three nights a week that's lasted for over a month. Your body and mind are aroused when you're trying to sleep, leading to a cycle of poor sleep and negative thoughts and behaviour patterns.

The most common symptoms of insomnia are:

✦ Difficulty falling asleep – also known as 'onset insomnia'. This is the most common sleep problem. For some people it can take a long time to drop off, but once they do their quality of sleep is good.
✦ Difficulty staying asleep – aka 'middle insomnia', the second most common problem. This is characterised by frequent waking in the middle of the night and then difficulty getting back to sleep.
✦ Waking up too early in the morning and not being able to drop off again.
✦ Unsatisfactory sleep quality. Some people sleep lightly, with restless, disturbed and inconsistent sleep. They'll feel irritable, tired and find it hard to function the next day.

It's important to rule out circumstances where these symptoms could be the result of any kind of drug, medication or medical condition (e.g. narcolepsy or generalised anxiety disorder).

The good news is there are proactive things you can do to combat everything from regular, but sporadic bad sleep to full-blown insomnia.

What makes us sleep?

There are two processes that work together to regulate our sleep:

✦ The sleep homeostat which controls our drive for sleep
✦ The circadian timer which controls when we sleep

The sleep homeostat: The word 'homeostasis' derives from the Greek word 'homeo' which means 'constant', and 'stasis' which means 'stable'. It describes a complex series of processes in the body that keeps our bodies both (yes, you guessed it) constant and stable. The sleep homeostat dictates how much sleep we need, dependent on how much sleep we've had and how tired we feel. For example, if you only snatch a couple of hours' sleep, your homeostat will make you feel sluggish, telling you to get some kip pronto to balance everything out and keep your body running smoothly. Think of it as an internal debt collector or regulator – you owe your body some sleep and your sleep homeostat is in charge of making sure you pay up.

The circadian timer: This is a fancy name for your body clock. Your body is programmed to respond to light and darkness in a twenty-four hour day and night cycle. Everyone's body clock is set slightly differently – you might be someone who's at their best in the morning, while others thrive in the afternoon or evening. It's all governed by the 'sleeping hormone' melatonin. When it's dark your brain instructs your pineal gland to secrete more melatonin which makes you feel tired, while less melatonin is released when it's light so you feel more awake. This is why shift workers and people who live in places with long dark winters (such as Scandinavian countries) can suffer from Seasonal

Affective Disorder (SAD). They'll produce more melatonin than usual or than is ideal (considering they need to work), leading to constant tiredness which can make them feel low emotionally. It's the reason – combined with the cold – that many of us feel the desire to 'hibernate' in the winter months, feeling unmotivated about venturing out in the darker evenings.

Sleep debt

Sleep debt is a simple way of thinking about what happens when you lose sleep. The more in debt you are (i.e. the more sleep you're not getting over time), the more tired you'll feel. The good news is that your sleep homeostat (debt collector) won't demand you catch up on all the hours you've missed immediately. You can pay them back the next night, over the next couple of weeks or even the next few months. This is a key reason why you shouldn't panic if you have a bad night or bad couple of nights sporadically. Research shows that even getting as little as two hours' sleep is enough to prevent detrimental effects on brain functioning – as long as this is only for the odd night here and there. You won't be on best form, but you'll manage just fine. The key thing to remember here is that getting less sleep occasionally is manageable, it's when it becomes frequent that it becomes a problem.

And there's more good news: you actually only need to make up one-third of the hours you've missed to get back to feeling your best. For example, if Lucy needs six hours' sleep a night to feel good, yet has only managed to get three hours for the last two nights she only needs to make up two of the six hours she's lost (one-third of the debt) and there's no deadline in which she needs to pay those hours back.

Your body compensates for what you've lost and will strike a balance between what you're getting and what you need.

The effects of not sleeping

The effects of regular sleeplessness can be, to put it bluntly, catastrophic. It can affect how you think and behave, and how you feel both emotionally and physically. These negative feelings and behaviours aren't just confined to night time; they'll spill into your day life as you worry about how you're going to cope with your responsibilities, even if, in reality, you'll cope just fine.

Physically, you can feel tired and achy, numb and disorientated. Also you might become clumsy as your reflexes slow down, affecting your hand and eye coordination. A research study looking at the links between sleep and physical health found that insomniacs were more likely to suffer from heart disease, high blood pressure, neurological disease, chronic pain and breathing, urinary and digestive issues. Great, eh?

Losing sleep can become all you think about. You'll worry about how you're performing now or how you're going to perform in the future, leaving you trying to anticipate and control sleep. If you're stressed at work or home this can snowball into a fear about not sleeping and often it's easier to make sleep the main focus of your concern rather than trying to deal with complicated life events. Your priorities get screwed up – you're trying to solve the sleeping problem rather than the original issue, not realising you're just putting yourself under more pressure and actively prolonging both problems. Your memory will suffer as you won't have processed information overnight and your thoughts can become jumbled up as you'll be easily distracted.

Emotionally, not sleeping can make you feel very low. You'll feel frustrated, scared, lonely and you'll start to wonder if things will ever improve. You can become snappy and moody, feeling anxious about how this is affecting you and what you can do about it.

Finally, lack of sleep can have a huge impact on your behaviour. You might start missing work or social events, feeling as if you can't cope with what's expected of you. This can affect your family, friends or partner, and your job. You might start changing your routine by introducing naps into your day or by avoiding going to bed until the early hours – all of which will only maintain your sleeplessness and perhaps even make it worse.

When you're in this state your body clock doesn't work properly – you're so preoccupied with sleep and the consequences of not getting enough that you've scuppered the natural, automatic process behind it all. The more you want and crave it, the more elusive sleep will become – it loves to play hard to get.

What affects your sleep?
Age
Age trumps absolutely everything in the sleep game. Newborns sleep pretty much non-stop, waking only to feed, while adolescents need less, but still a fair amount (teenagers aren't just lazy sods). Then, as you get older you need less and less sleep and the sort of sleep you get changes. You're no longer physically growing so your body doesn't demand the same amount or intensity of rest time. As you reach old age, your sleep will become lighter and more broken, you'll start dropping off during the day and sleep for less time during the night.

The vicious circle of sleep deprivation

Can't fall asleep, can't stay asleep, or keep waking very early

Feel physically achy, tired and clumsy

Think 'I can't cope with no sleep'/ 'This will never get any better'

Feel low, anxious, frustrated and irritable

Start avoiding going to bed or having naps during the day

Lifestyle and environment

Your surroundings and environment can have a huge effect on your sleep. This includes being too hot or too cold, your room being too light or too noisy, being somewhere new, or sleeping next to someone whose snores rattle the windows. Diet, exercise and the hours you work will also have an impact.

Stress, anxiety and emotional upheaval

If you're stressed and worrying about something going on in your life (or about sleep itself) you'll find it harder to drop off. Major life events both positive (e.g. getting married or getting a new job) and negative (e.g. financial stress, divorce or grief) can all leave you either lying awake at night or waking up up in the early hours.

Physical health

Trying to sleep with a blocked nose, earache or a bad back is often ridiculous. You can't breathe or move for pain so how are you meant to sleep? Long-term conditions such as osteoporosis or diabetes can drastically mess with your sleeping patterns. Addressing your physical health issues can have the knock-on effect of solving your sleeping problems. As we mentioned in the introduction if you believe you may be suffering from sleep apnoea (a temporary pause in breathing while sleeping), sleepwalking or restless leg syndrome you should contact your GP. However, if it's snoring that's keeping you awake, 99 per cent of all cases can be cured by simple over-the-counter remedies.

Mental health

Sleeping badly can increase the risk of a mental health problem or be one of the symptoms of a mental health problem – it goes both ways. If you believe you may be suffering from a psychological disorder such as depression, generalised anxiety disorder or post-traumatic stress disorder then please visit your GP as well as carrying on working through this book. With depression it is important to work out if your sleep issues are a consequence of your mood or vice versa. If you think your sleep problems might be a symptom of depression it's essential you seek out appropriate treatment. A combination approach to both your sleeping problem and your mental health problem is essential so the strategies we recommend will help.

Recognising yourself in any of the above (or perhaps in all of the above) is positive, believe it or not, because there are simple and effective ways of dealing with most of these issues (apart from getting older – sorry – but you can encourage better sleeping patterns no matter how old you are). However, even if you can't see any obvious reason for your sleep problems, changing what you do and how you think and feel about sleep will help enormously.

Other things that affect sleep
Dreaming

No one really understands dreams. They might claim to, but they don't really. There is no definitive data that can break down what they are, where they come from and why we have them. Some scientists believe they serve no real purpose, while others reckon they're integral to our mental, emotional and physical well-being (yes, that's how varied the theories get). Freud believed dreams are subconscious representations of your innermost desires – an attempt by your unconscious to identify and resolve important thoughts, wishes and problems that your conscious mind will have to deal with later. Whether you choose to believe this or not is completely up to you; all we know scientifically is that dreams are associated with the chemical dopamine. Dopamine is a neurotransmitter (a chemical that transmits signals within the brain) that plays a part in deciding what we should concentrate on – it can bring things to the fore or push them to the back. The part of the brain that deals with emotions, sensations and memories becomes more active during the stage of sleep where you're most likely to dream (this is the REM stage which we discuss in more detail later on), so it could be that the brain makes sense of this internal activity by creating dreams – movies in your head. Another theory suggests that dreams may help you maintain sleep by keeping the mind occupied so that you don't wake up while other parts of your brain are resting and recovering. These are all just theories though – feel free to add some of your own.

Nightmares

Nightmares are hideous, but everyone gets them occasionally. The official definition is 'an intense frightening dream that wakes the sleeper in a panicked state'. Usually nightmares occur in the early morning and they are often influenced by uncomfortable experiences or thoughts that happened the previous day. Recurrent nightmares (i.e. repeatedly dreaming you're running as fast as you can, but not actually moving anywhere) are believed to be the result of anxiety. Following a terrible dream you can experience an episode of sleep paralysis if you wake suddenly. Your muscles are paralysed during REM sleep and they can remain paralysed for a short time if you wake up in shock.

Night terrors

Night terrors are, well, terrifying. They're a disruption to sleep where you wake up feeling uncontrollable fear and panic. Your heart rate rockets and you may sweat and even scream. They're far more dramatic than nightmares as they only happen during very deep sleep and aren't caused by dreams – it's a purely emotional response triggered by nothing specific. The good news is that you won't remember anything the next day as you weren't dreaming so there won't be any toe-curling images to recall. Normally night terrors begin and end in childhood. Approximately 18 per cent of children experience them, but only about 2 per cent of the adult population. Night terrors are more likely to occur when sleep deprived, after drinking alcohol or during a period of stress. Night terrors in adults are usually associated with a previous trauma so if this sounds like something you can relate to you should see your GP.

Sleepwalking and sleep talking

These occur during deep sleep, they're not related to dreaming and people rarely remember doing it when they wake up (very annoying for witnesses). Sleepwalking is most common in children between the ages of five to twelve years. 15 per cent of children are said to walk in their sleep at least once. It is much less common in adults, occurring in about 2–5 per cent of the adult population, the majority of whom began sleepwalking when they were children. Like night terrors, they're more likely to occur when you are sleep deprived, have been drinking alcohol or feeling stressed. Sleep talking occurs in about 4 per cent of adults (again it's more common in children). It can range from non-verbal utterances to eloquent speeches, but is rarely a serious problem for the speaker – more so for the partner.

Teeth grinding (also known as sleep bruxism)

About 8 per cent of the general population are estimated to grind their teeth at least twice a week at night. It's more common in people who consume large amounts of caffeine, alcohol and nicotine and can be symptomatic of underlying stress and anxiety. It not only disrupts your sleep, but can give you jaw ache and headaches and even damage your teeth. For long-term grinding problems it's important to take steps to deal with any stress or anxiety in your life and consider visiting your dentist who might be able to fashion you a mouth guard to protect your teeth.

The simple act of not being able to sleep can have devastating consequences, but changing how you think, behave and feel about it can actually solve the problem. This is where Cognitive Behavioural Therapy (CBT) comes in (see Chapter 2).

Thoughts to take away

✓ Changing how you feel and think about sleep will alter how well you sleep

✓ There are proactive things you can do to improve your chances of dropping off and sleeping through the night

✓ You can't force sleep, but you can encourage it by stopping bad habits

2

Cognitive Behavioural Therapy

Cognitive Behavioural Therapy (CBT) provides techniques to change how you think, feel and react to sleep. Here we explain why it's brilliant and how it will help *you*.

What is CBT?

Cognitive Behavioural Therapy might sound like an evaluation you'd undergo before boarding the Starship Enterprise, but thankfully it's nothing of the sort. Pioneered by Dr Aaron T. Beck in the 1960s and recommended by the National Institute of Clinical Excellence (NICE), CBT is one of the leading treatments for a wide variety of disorders including depression, anxiety, OCD (obsessive compulsive disorder) and yes, insomnia. It gives you control when you feel most out of control by teaching you practical strategies to manage your day-to-day (and night-to-night) life. And once you have these tools they'll stay with you forever so you can fall back on them whenever you need to.

CBT is one of the most widely used and successful therapies for sleep problems and will improve your ability to get to sleep, limit the times you wake up during the night, help you sleep for longer, and generally make going to bed less of an ordeal. Reports by the American Academy of Sleep Medicine show that across eighty-five clinical trials, CBT helped over two-thirds of patients.

Best of all, CBT is time-efficient. You're not starting treatment that will drag on for years – it's all about feeling better now, no matter what's happened to you in the past. If you really throw yourself into it, you'll be sleeping better in a matter of weeks.

The fundamental principle behind CBT is this: how you interpret a situation or perceive an event will affect your thoughts, your behaviour and how you feel physically and emotionally. You construct a belief about what's going on around you and then act on it.

For example, Dan has a terrible night's sleep, writhing around worrying about the big presentation he has to give at work tomorrow.

He wakes up after dropping off for only an hour and immediately thinks, 'I'm too tired to handle today.' This thought leaves him feeling anxious and questioning his ability to cope. He also feels angry because this just had to happen to him today of all days, didn't it? Dan tenses up physically and notices a nervous twitch in his eye. He worries whether colleagues will notice his fatigue so informs everyone about his sleep issues. Rather than helping the situation though, this makes people question whether he's up to the task. The fact he didn't sleep has become the thing Dan's focusing on, rather than the presentation itself – which will no doubt have a detrimental effect on how he performs.

Compare that to Louise. She's got an interview with the CEO of a company she's always wanted to work for tomorrow. It's her dream job and she's down to the final two. She doesn't get any sleep the night before – she can't stop practising all her answers to the questions she thinks she'll be asked. When she gets up she feels physically weary, but is pumped full of adrenaline. She feels excited and nervous and doesn't let her sleepiness affect her behaviour at all. She thinks, 'I'm tired, but I can do this. I just need to get through the day and I'll catch up on my sleep tonight when the interview's over.'

CBT will teach you to start examining what you do, how you feel both emotionally and physically and to start questioning your thoughts and their validity. By making some fundamental changes to how you interpret situations you'll be able to stop your sleeping patterns ruling your life. For example, when you next have trouble sleeping and anxiety, worry and self-criticism kick in, instead of reacting like Dan, stop, take a moment and consciously choose to reassure and encourage yourself like Louise. So, rather than hearing a miserable and panicky voice in your head you'll be hearing a compassionate motivator reminding you that everything is going to be okay and that one bad night's sleep isn't the end of the world. This will make you feel more in

Example: Lydia's lie-in

Lydia was on a sun, sea and sangria holiday with a group of friends. They spent every day camped on the beach reading, chatting and listening to music, before moving on to the local bars in the evening. It should have been exactly what she needed after a horribly stressful couple of months at work. Except it wasn't.

Every night they'd return to their hotel in the early hours and everyone else would fall asleep immediately and stay that way until mid-morning. Apart from Lydia. She tossed and turned or stared at the ceiling thinking, 'If I don't sleep the whole holiday will be ruined.' No matter how tired she was and how much she craved sleep she just couldn't drop off. Then at about 8a.m. she'd snatch a couple of hours before being woken up by her friends.

After three consecutive nights of this, Lydia felt irritable and exhausted. She skipped the next two evenings out because she thought she'd be bad company. She watched bad telly instead and began to feel angry and panicky about whether she'd ever be able to sleep normally again.

control of your thoughts which, coupled with the positive stuff you'll be hearing, will make you feel more confident. Changing how you think about sleep will have a positive impact on how you feel and what you do.

Lydia's mind map

We've explained what happened to Lydia in a snazzy diagram called a mind map.

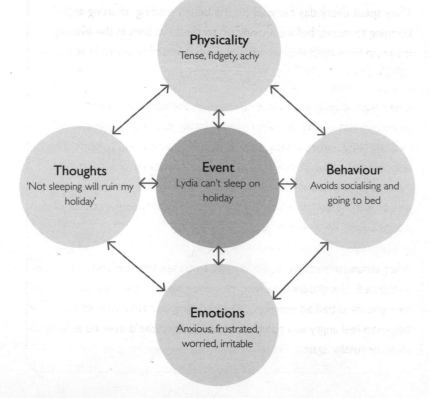

Physicality
Tense, fidgety, achy

Thoughts
'Not sleeping will ruin my holiday'

Event
Lydia can't sleep on holiday

Behaviour
Avoids socialising and going to bed

Emotions
Anxious, frustrated, worried, irritable

Mind maps are designed to show the links between how you think, how you behave and how you feel emotionally and physically. Lydia's negative thoughts triggered a tense reaction in her body which made her act in a way she wouldn't normally (avoiding socialising), which made her feel low and anxious. However, it could have been her physical response that set everything else off – her aching and tense body prompting her to act out of character, influencing her thoughts and her mood.

Your body, your thoughts and your behaviour can all act as intervention points – change these and the rest will follow like dominoes, which will lift your mood. If Lydia had thought, 'It doesn't really matter if I get lots of sleep because I'm not doing anything stressful,' instead of, 'This is going to ruin the trip,' her body wouldn't have tensed up at night, she wouldn't have felt anxious and she wouldn't have stayed behind while her friends went out. Because her mind and body were all riled up she physically couldn't get to sleep.

Stepping back and interpreting things in a objective and realistic way will not only make you feel better, but will actually help you get to sleep as both your mind and body become more relaxed.

Ⓢ Your own mind map

Now you know a bit more about CBT, you can fill in your own mind map. Start by identifying a recent, well remembered situation you experienced concerning sleep, e.g. not being able to get to sleep, waking up early or tossing and turning. Then work through the four points in the circles in whatever order comes naturally to you:

Your interpretive options

CBT will show you that there are choices when it comes to how you interpret what happens. If you can't sleep you can think:

'This always happens to me' → depressed
'I'll be too tired to cope with tomorrow' → anxious
'This is so unfair!' → angry
'I'll manage' → calm

The last option is far more likely to lead to a positive outcome – both in your day-to-day life and when you go to bed.

1 **Thoughts:** When you were in the situation, what went through your mind (your stand-out thought)?
2 **Emotions:** How did you feel emotionally? Anxious, frustrated, angry?
3 **Physicality:** How did you feel physically e.g. tense, increased heart rate, sweating?
4 **Behaviour:** What action did you take or think about taking?

When you've filled it in evaluate what you've discovered. Can you see the link between all four points? Which section did you find easiest to fill in? Do you tend to experience sleeplessness physically first or mentally? Exploring your reactions to sleep will allow you to question what's actually happening and to look for alternative ways of thinking, feeling and behaving – ways that'll have a more positive chain-reaction.

Sleeping: a bit of a nightmare

Even good sleepers can experience problems at various points in their lives, usually if they have something on their minds. Take Dan and Louise above – they were both thinking about specific events when they should have been sleeping. If you have a stressful event coming up (either a negative or a positive one) you might find your sleep disrupted because your brain will be more alert than usual, trying to process everything that's going on. Chances are that when the event is over your sleep will revert back to normal. However, this isn't always the case. Often when your sleeping patterns change – no matter how briefly – you worry about it, over-think it and change your routine to try to compensate for it (i.e. taking naps or drinking alcohol before you go to bed). This can exacerbate the issue so it doesn't disappear along with the problem that triggered it. Sleep has now become the issue rather than a symptom of the original issue.

Your body can get into a routine of not sleeping whenever you're stressed and then your negative thoughts, emotions and behavioural patterns kick in, which only serve to maintain the problem. How you think, feel and behave when you're tired during the day and when you're trying to drop off will all have a big influence on sleep.

Common thoughts, feelings and behaviours linked to lack of sleep

Over-thinking sleep

When you can't sleep it'll clog up your brain, sucking up all your thoughts. You'll start trying to control something that is supposed to be as automatic as breathing. You'll mark your nights as either successes or failures: 'I got three hours last night which is the worst this week – fail!' You're putting yourself under more and more pressure to succeed which will have exactly the opposite effect. Thinking about not sleeping makes it a self-fulfilling prophecy – you're thinking about it while you should be doing it! Night time becomes a trial to be endured rather than a time to recharge and rest.

Physical and emotional reactions

When you're stressed and anxious you'll tense up physically. Your fight or flight response kicks in – a hangover from our cave-dwelling days – and your body goes into 'attack mode'. The hormones adrenaline and cortisol flood your system making your muscles tense, your heart race, body sweat and blood flood the areas of your body and brain that need it most. All of which is great if you're battling a woolly mammoth, but not so great if you're trying to relax and get to sleep. You're scared of not sleeping, yet all your body recognises is the feeling of fear – not the cause behind it. This can leave you feeling physically exhausted the next day.

Behaving badly

A lack of sleep can influence your behaviour in two ways – both in your 'day life' and in your 'night life'. It can make you act out of character during the day, because you're sluggish and can't concentrate e.g. you'll snap at people or start drinking lots of coffee to try to perk yourself up. And it can make you change your behaviour when you're trying to sleep – e.g. by spending too long in bed tossing and turning or by taking sleeping pills. By trying to control how you sleep you're fundamentally altering your sleep homeostat and circadian rhythm, making it harder to return to a natural sleep process.

Symptoms checklist

Now you have a better idea how your sleeping patterns are being messed up, it's time to start thinking about why. Have a look at the tick boxes below and mark off any that ring true for you.

Emotions

❑ Stressed: Under pressure
❑ Anxious: Fearful about future events
❑ Irritable

❑ Frustrated
❑ Low/ sad/ miserable
❑ Depressed
❑ Quickly changing moods

Physically

❑ Feeling weary during the day
❑ Clumsy
❑ Body feels stiff
❑ Poor concentration and a low attention span
❑ Tense

❑ Headaches
❑ Upset stomach/digestive problems
❑ Slow reflexes
❑ Disorientated

Thoughts

❑ Constantly thinking about not sleeping

❑ Worrying about other problems and stresses apart from sleeping

❑ Thinking about your past day and upcoming day (not necessarily negatively)

❑ Waking up worrying and not being able to return to sleep

❑ Impaired judgement in your day life due to lack of sleep

❑ Sluggish and more negative day-to-day thoughts

❑ Being forgetful

Behaviour

❑ Avoiding socialising

❑ Staying up late to avoid going to bed

❑ Being snappy with friends, colleagues, family members

❑ Creating conflict in relationships

❑ Drinking more alcohol

❑ Taking recreational drugs

❑ Taking medicinal drugs (self-medicating)

❑ Napping

❑ Taking time off work

❑ Making mistakes at work or home

By recognising how what you're thinking, doing and feeling is all influencing, and being influenced by, how you sleep you're giving yourself more opportunities to get out of the no-sleep rut. Changing one aspect of your life for the better will have a knock-on effect with the others, altering how you think and feel about sleep – and ultimately how you sleep.

⑤ Thoughts aren't facts

This is an integral message of CBT and something we'll bang on about throughout the book. It's amazing how often we just accept something that we've thought of as a truth without challenging it or acknowledging how damaging it might be. For example, 'No one likes to be around me when I'm tired.' You're telling this to yourself as if it's a fact, when in reality it's complete nonsense. Unless you've actually asked everybody whether or not they like you when you're tired, there's no way you could know this for certain.

You may view these thoughts as inconsequential, but this couldn't be further from the truth. As you'll know from this chapter, your thoughts influence how you feel emotionally and physically, and how you behave. That tiny thought could make you feel despondent, which will make your body tense up leading you to snap at a colleague, giving you something else to worry about – all of which will stop you sleeping. These thoughts matter.

When you think something it's just a thought – a hypothesis, an opinion. You have to acknowledge and accept this so the next time a distressing thought pops into your head masquerading as a fact you can challenge it. Is this true? No? Then dismiss it.

Example: Mark's dozing dramas

Mark hadn't been sleeping well for a couple of months. Every time he got into bed his mind started reeling – replaying everything that had happened that day and everything that might happen tomorrow. He wasn't under a particular amount of stress, but the lack of sleep was starting to make him feel drained and agitated.

Mark's thoughts:
Theory A: 'I'll never sleep normally again'
Theory B: 'I think I'll never sleep normally again'

The difference between Mark's two theories is huge. In theory A he's stating an unrealistic fearful thought as if it's fact. The chances that he'll never sleep normally again are slim to none. There are loads of proactive things he can do to provoke positive sleeping patterns (like reading this book of course). This thought will have whizzed through his brain unacknowledged and gone on to create a negative sequence of events all based upon something that isn't true.

By thinking this way, Mark is not giving himself a chance to challenge this thought. Whereas, by taking a step back and going for theory B he's recognising that there's room for manoeuvre. He can work out when he did last have a good night's sleep and what he did differently then. Also, he'll be able to acknowledge ⋯⋮

⋯⋮ that there are things he can do to encourage a normal sleeping routine.

When people think more realistically they feel more in control – less panicked and stressed – which will make dealing with sleeping problems easier and less intimidating.

Next steps ...

CBT starts by asking you to look at your behaviour around sleep – how what you do might be stopping you from getting the sleep you need. Behaviour is an easy one to start with as you can make immediate changes. You'll then automatically feel better emotionally because you're taking positive action and not floundering in a red-eyed sleepless abyss.

CBT aims to:

+ Help you change your sleeping environment so it's more conducive to sleep
+ Stop unhelpful behaviours that reduce your chances of sleeping
+ Teach you relaxation and wind-down techniques
+ Combat negative thoughts about sleep and test out alternative interpretations
+ Learn strategies and techniques to help you manage and reduce stress
+ Renew the positive association between your bed and sleep

CBT is an active approach to solving problems in your life – you'll need to really throw yourself into the strategies. Doing things differently will change how you feel and think about sleep and ultimately how well you sleep.

Thoughts to take away

✓ You can change how you think and feel about sleep and your sleeping habits

✓ Sleep isn't the enemy so stop treating it like one

✓ Recognise that thoughts aren't facts!

3

Sleep Myths Laid to Rest

Now you know a bit more about *why* you sleep, we're moving on to how you sleep. Monitoring your own sleep will force you to acknowledge what's actually happening, to face your fears and to confront that elusive sandman.

The sleep cycle

There are five different stages of sleep and the process is cyclical.
You'll go through each of the five stages more than once a night and
typically wake up a few times too. Waking up intermittently is totally
normal – it's part and parcel of the lighter stages of sleep, a genetic
tick from prehistoric days when our senses were on high alert all the
time, sensitive to any possible danger. It's why you'll jolt awake if you
hear something that could be construed as threatening no matter how
deeply asleep you are, and also why a new mother will instinctively
hear her baby whimpering nearby.

The first four stages of sleep are called non-rapid eye movement
sleep (NREM) while the fifth is called (surprise, surprise) rapid eye
movement sleep (REM). The names are self-explanatory: in stages 1–4
your eyes don't move, while in 5 they do – but that's by far the least
interesting aspect of what's going on.

During a single night you may experience four or five recurring
sleep cycles, each cycle lasting between 70–120 minutes. The length
of the cycles increases towards the end of the night, averaging at about
90–120 minutes, however you won't necessarily experience each stage
during each cycle. For example, on your third and fourth cycles you
might miss out stage 4 – the deepest sleep stage – going straight from
stage 3 to 5, like jumping gears in a car. Deep sleep typically happens at
the start of sleep and occupies less time or even disappears altogether
in the later cycles.

The five stages of sleep

NREM (non-rapid eye movement sleep) occurs for approximately 75 per cent of the time you're asleep and is broken down into four stages:

+ **Stage 1:** The stage between sleep and wakefulness when you've almost dropped off, but not quite. Have you ever woken up and turned on the light because of a suspicious shadow, sat up because you're convinced you heard someone calling your name or experienced a falling sensation before jerking awake? That will all happen in stage 1, the lightest stage of sleep, when dreams can seem to merge with reality. Your muscle movement slows down and you may twitch – which annoyingly can also wake you.

+ **Stage 2:** The onset of sleep. You'll become disengaged from your surroundings and less aware of the outside world. Your body temperature will drop and your breathing and heart rate will slow down. This is still considered relatively light sleep, yet accounts for 45–50 per cent of all sleep in adults.

+ **Stages 3 and 4:** The last stages of NREM sleep are typically lumped together, as stage 3 is a transition platform into stage 4. These are the deepest and most restorative parts of sleep, known as 'delta sleep' or 'synchronised sleep'. Stage 4 boasts the lordly title of 'true delta' and is responsible for giving your body time to start restoring and resting itself. Your blood pressure drops, your breathing and heart rate reach their lowest, most rhythmic levels and blood rushes to your now completely relaxed muscles to aid tissue growth and repair. Growth hormones flood your system (more so in kids and teenagers) while your brain starts consolidating what it's learned during the day, filing stuff away like an efficient secretary. If woken up during this stage you'll feel shocked, groggy and disoriented for several minutes.

REM sleep is the fifth stage – the last part of the cycle before it starts all over again. It accounts for 25 per cent of your sleep.

+ **Stage 5:** This takes its name from the rapid eye movements that the sleeper undergoes, (usually with their eyes closed – but not always!), as discovered in 1953 by Nathaniel Kleitman and Eugene Aserinsky. The frequency of one's rapid eye movements is known as their REM density. During this stage, the brainwaves are similar to when we are resting.

This type of sleep is characterised by electrical activation of the brain which causes your eyes to dart rapidly back and forth under closed eyelids. While dreams can occur during any of the five stages, they're more likely to happen now and it's thought your eyes move because you're following images from your dreams – watching a movie in your head.

Your eyes aren't actually sending any visual data to your brain, but studies have shown that the visual cortex – the part of the brain that processes images – is active. It is doing something, just what though is not clearly understood. Scientists believe it might be part of a memory-forming or memory-reinforcing process where your mind files away everything that happened during the day. Cleverly though, messages from your brain paralyse your muscles so you can't try to act out your dreams. This is a relatively shallow stage of sleep, your breathing rate and blood pressure rise and your brain polishes up all your memories and dusts off your concentration, leaving you ready for the day ahead. The average person will have three to five episodes of REM sleep per night, with the first likely to begin about 70–90 minutes after falling asleep.

To wake up feeling refreshed and as un-zombie-like as possible you need to spend enough time in each of the stages during the night, which typically works out something like this:

Stage 1: 5 per cent of the night
Stage 2: 50 per cent
Stage 3 and 4: 20 per cent
Stage 5: 25 per cent

All of which is handily explained in the diagram below:

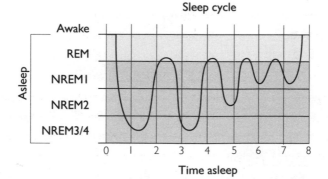

Sleep cycle

While you're asleep

Exceptionally important things happen to your body while you're asleep:

+ **Brain maintenance:** The brain's cerebral cortex has a rest and repairs itself, ensuring your memories are intact, your mind's functioning as it should, and your body is undertaking all the repair, growth and development it needs.

+ **Repair:** Your body goes into repair mode when you sleep, regenerating skin, muscles, blood and brain cells. Getting enough sleep can hugely affect your appearance which is why it's called 'beauty sleep'. Glowing skin and no bags under your eyes are signs of a good night's rest. More worryingly, new studies have shown a lack of sleep elevates substances in the blood responsible for increasing inflammation in the body leading to an increased risk of heart disease, cancer, strokes, diabetes and obesity.

+ **Blood pressure control:** When you sleep your blood pressure drops which moderates levels during the day too.

+ **Weight control:** Research has found that sleep disruption raises blood levels of ghrelin, a hormone linked to feeling hungry, and decreases levels of leptin, the hormone that tells you you're full. Not only is your body physically encouraging you to eat ⋯⋮

⋯ more if you're tired, but mentally you'll be more tempted to reach for high-sugar snacks to boost your energy levels. If you feel sluggish you're less likely to be active and burn those extra calories off. On top of all that, your metabolism slows down when you're sleep deprived, meaning you're more likely to put on weight.

+ **Immune system restoration:** Your immune system restores and detoxifies. Sleeplessness can make you more susceptible to illness.

Sleeping with one eye open

We've already covered how there is no such thing as a generic 'perfect' night's sleep – everyone needs different things. That whole 'falling asleep as soon as your head hits the pillow' shtick can be very damaging if you're using it as a measure of what should be happening when you go to bed. Good sleepers generally take approximately fifteen minutes to fall asleep and will wake up at least once during the night during the lighter sleep stages. If you're expecting to drop off as soon as you get in bed and then leap up exactly eight hours later, you're going to be sorely disappointed. Don't put unnecessary pressure on yourself based upon unrealistic standards.

Some people are just gifted at sleeping, just like some people are gifted at painting or playing tennis. It's a natural skill. However, just like painting and tennis you can improve your ability to sleep by practising different techniques and approaches, which is where our anti-lethargy lessons come in.

Anti-lethargy lessons

These are the lessons you need to learn and adopt into your day-to-day life. They're truths that people with sleep problems often forget, don't know or refuse to believe. Accepting these will lift a huge weight off your shoulders as you realise you can learn to sleep better, there's no definitive one-size-fits-all when it comes to sleep and you don't have to panic when things don't go according to plan.

+ There is not a 'perfect' amount of sleep appropriate for everyone. This key fact should stop you trying to force yourself to conform to a spurious ideal.

+ Don't compare how you sleep (i.e. deeply, immediately, intermittently) to others – everyone is different.

+ Your sleep needs will vary over time and in different situations i.e. you might need more when you're working particularly hard, but you can get by on less when you need to (i.e when you've had a baby).

+ There are lots of factors that contribute to how well you function – sleep is just one of them. Your body will try to deal with whatever's thrown at it no matter how little sleep you've had. As easy as it might be to pin a bad mood or bad behaviour on sleeplessness there will definitely be other triggers. Even good sleepers get grumpy and make mistakes sometimes. ⋯⋰

⋯⫶

+ How much sleep you need might be different from how much
  sleep you want, i.e. you might want to get by on four hours a night,
  but in reality need seven or eight. Your body will ensure that what
  you need will always take priority so it's best to accept this now
  and work from there.

⑤ Your anti-lethargy mind map

Pick one of the anti-lethargy lessons above and really embrace it for a day and night. Choose the one that most strikes a chord with you. If you're worried about how sleeplessness is affecting you during the day, make this your twenty-four-hour mantra: 'there are lots of factors that contribute to how well you function – sleep is just one of them'. This should reassure you that your body and mind will work out a way to get you through the day no matter how shattered you are.

Repeat the lesson to yourself until you know it off by heart and set it as a reminder on your phone to go off every hour or couple of hours. It's all very well just reading this stuff, but you have to choose to actively accept it. These lessons will make you feel more positive about sleep, which will, in turn, make it easier to get to sleep.

Example: Mike's midnight madness/Mike's new mantra

Mike had recently found himself getting incensed by his girlfriend's ability to just hop into bed and be dead to the world within minutes. Her rhythmic breaths had become the backing track for his angry tossing and turning. Her ability to sleep was actually aggravating his inability to sleep. He found himself timing how quickly it took her to start snoozing in comparison with how long it took him to drop off.

He picked the anti-lethargy lesson 'there is not a "perfect" amount of sleep appropriate for everyone' and set it to ping up on his phone on the hour during the day. That night he went to bed feeling less tense about the prospect of lying next to his conked-out girlfriend. He'd been okay on the hours he'd been getting – he hadn't been at his best, but he'd managed – so perhaps trying to get as much sleep as her was counter-productive? When they got into bed that night he read his book rather than staring at the ceiling. An hour later he turned off the light. Half an hour after that he was asleep.

Mike took control of how he thought and felt about sleep. Instead of panicking about being awake longer than his girlfriend he just accepted it, so when he did finally drop off he slept more soundly. His mind map looked like this (see opposite).

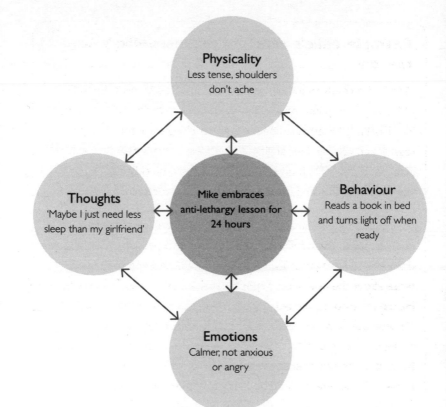

Now it's your turn. Fill in your own mind map after spending twenty-four hours imbibing an anti-lethargy lesson. How did it make you feel, think and behave? This is all about taking control of how you deal with sleep. You can't control the act itself, but you can put a plan in place to control how you respond to it.

Sleep monitoring

Everyone's susceptible to a bit of exaggeration when they've had a bad night – 'I didn't sleep a wink,' or 'I only slept for an hour'. The trouble is, this isn't just a case of sympathy pandering or good story-telling, we're all fairly rubbish at estimating how long we've been asleep for and how sound that sleep was.

Research has found that compared to normal sleepers, insomniacs hugely underestimate how long they've been snoozing and are more likely to report they've only just dropped off if they're woken up after their first sleep cycle (which on average lasts between 70–120 minutes). It's why you'll shout, 'What? I wasn't asleep!' when your partner jabs you in the ribs for snoring.

It's really important to find out how much sleep you're actually getting and how much you need. And remember: there is no golden standard of sleep that works for everyone. The following strategies will allow you to discover what's really happening with your sleep.

⑤ Your mini sleep assessment

It's important to review your sleeping patterns – to really think about them in detail and not just dismiss them as 'generally hopeless'.

Answer the questions below:

1 Trying to be as specific as you can:
   + When did your sleep problem(s) first start?
   + What was/were the trigger(s)?
   + Have there been other periods in your life when you have slept poorly?

2 How long have you had poor sleep (both this time and any previous times)?
  + Frequency (once a year/once a month, etc.)
  + Severity (how bad do you judge the problem to be?)
  + Duration (how long does each bout last?)

3 How does poor sleep affect you?
  + Look back at the boxes you ticked in the symptoms checklist in Chapter 2 and note down which most concern you and which ones prompted you to pick up this book

There are no right or wrong answers – this is an exercise to get you thinking about what's actually happening and what you want to change. If you've always been a terrible sleeper suddenly aiming for eight hours a night is unrealistic and probably unnecessary. Also, filling in the mini assessment may have made you realise that this bout of troubled sleep is exactly the same as the one you had a couple of years ago, when you were also going through a major life change. From there you can start thinking about how you managed previously and what eventually stopped the problem. Stepping back from the issue will give you an objectivity that can be hard to summon when you're exhausted and frustrated.

⑤ Your sleep diary

Welcome to your sleep diary! You'll need to keep this every week throughout the process. It's simple to follow and some of the later strategies we'll suggest rely on the information gleaned from filling it in. Make it part of your morning routine – the amount of effort you put in now will pay dividends later.

First up, you need to find out exactly how long you're currently sleeping, rather than guessing. At the end of seven days you'll be able to identify which nights you slept better or worse, and from there work out what could be causing any problems, e.g. did you read your work emails one night or stay up late drinking? When the week is up you'll also be able to narrow down what your specific problem is: getting to sleep or staying asleep – or both. We have shown a column for Monday, so you can follow this and add the other days of the week.

Sleep experience	Monday
How well did you sleep last night? (1–10)	
What time did you fall asleep? (approx.)	
Roughly how long did it take you to fall asleep (from turning your light out to sleeping)?	
How many times did you wake in the night?	
How long were you awake throughout the night?	
What time did you wake up in the morning?	
How long did you sleep for in total?	
How well rested do you feel? (1–10)	
How well did you function during the day? (1–10)	
How was your mood during the day? (1–10)	
Any other comments Rating: 1 = awful, 10 = amazing	

After you've completed the week, assess what you've discovered. Were you surprised by any of the results? Perhaps you thought falling asleep was your biggest problem, but actually you felt much worse after the night you woke up six times. Or maybe you thought you were awake for most of the night, but in fact you got four hours' sleep.

Having your assumptions confirmed or disproved is a key part of thinking differently about sleep. Okay, so you did feel rubbish after only four hours' sleep – but maybe you actually functioned just about okay and then made the hours up later in the week.

Work out the average amount of sleep you got per night (total amount of hours per week divided by seven) – this is the baseline that we're going to work to improve.

Thoughts to take away

✓ There is no gold standard when it comes to sleep – everyone is different!

✓ You can train yourself to be 'better' at sleeping just like you can train yourself to be better at tennis

✓ Your sleep diary will confirm or disprove your assumptions about how you really sleep, leaving you better equipped to make positive changes

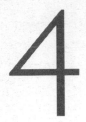

Wherever You Lay Your Head

Sleep is rather like a demanding house guest with very specific bedroom tastes (no, not *those* kinds of tastes). In this chapter we examine how to ensure the place you rest is actually conducive to sleep.

Haven or Hell

When you can't sleep your bedroom can become a place you dread – somewhere that invokes feelings of loneliness and fear. Like a prison cell – but with nicer curtains. Your mind and body react to your room negatively as any cues you once had associating it with sleep and relaxation have long-since disintegrated. You need to start re-associating your bedroom and your bed with the pleasures of sleep, rather than with frustration.

We've laid out some specific bedroom issues that might be contributing to rubbish sleep, along with great strategies for combating them. This process is part of Stimulus Control Therapy which is proven to strengthen the bed–sleep link. It's all about creating new cues in your bedroom to provoke a positive mental and physical response that's conducive to sleep rather than a 'get me out of here immediately' panic. Please note that it's crucial you take on board all the strategies whether you think you're susceptible to a problem or not. Lots of small changes will equal one massive difference to your life.

Danielle's discovery

Danielle reckoned she could sleep through anything. Storms? No problem. Parties? Easy. Fireworks? Whatever. She prided herself on her ability to drop off anywhere at any time. Or at least she did ... until she started suffering from insomnia. ⋯⋱

∙∙∙⫶∙ Sound, regular sleep became a distant memory as she lay awake for hours staring at the ceiling. However, she snorted derisively when someone suggested getting rid of the loud ticking clock in her bedroom as it might be disturbing her. She'd managed to sleep through years of her brother's heavy metal band rehearsing in a next-door bedroom: the clock definitely wasn't an issue. However, after another week of terrible sleep Danielle did move the clock just to see what would happen and she was shocked to find that it made a difference.

By altering the noise levels in her bedroom, she'd changed how she experienced the room and therefore felt more in control. Even though the noise itself didn't bother Danielle, doing something proactive altered how she viewed the room. This inspired her to try all the other strategies too and both her sleep and how she felt about it improved dramatically.

Because you can't control sleep you have to pick your battles – changing the environment you sleep in will make you feel you have some power over the situation.

After making the changes Danielle's mind map looked like this:

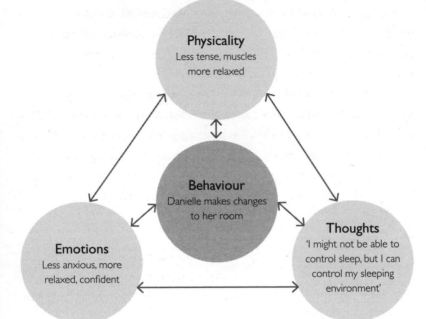

All of the little alterations we recommend will add up to a big difference. If you change everything that might be hindering your ability to sleep, your experience of your bedroom, bed and resting will be totally different, which can only be a good thing.

⑤ Battling the bedroom blues

Your bedroom needs to be welcoming and calming. Obviously we don't know your personal situation – you may share a bedroom or live in a studio where your bed is part of the main living area – but it doesn't matter. All the things we suggest can relate to any type of room.

You have a duty of care to yourself to make where you sleep somewhere you can actually relax. Good sleep is an essential part of your general health. You look after other aspects of your well-being so taking care of this part too makes sense.

Your bedroom should only be for sleeping and sex. (Getting dressed/ undressed is classed as an extension of the sleep process.) This should be the room you associate with sleep and sex and that's all. At the moment it might be the room you associate with lying awake and feeling anxious, meaning that you become tense and nervous as soon as you step inside – not a state conducive to sound sleep.

Ⓢ Your bedroom commandments

1 Own your room. Make it personal, somewhere you like to spend time. Put up photos that trigger happy memories, hang artwork you like, decorate it with throws and cushions. Make it your space rather than just a space.

2 Paint the walls neutral colours: whites, pale greys or creams. Blue and green are also calming and are proven to increase feelings of well-being, while bright reds, yellows and oranges are stimulating so are more likely to arouse your senses – not ideal when you're trying to drop off.

3 Invest in some room scent, incense or essential oils to dab onto your pillow. Walking into a room to a waft of chamomile, lavender, bergamot, jasmine, rose or sandalwood (all proven to induce a sense of calm) will make you feel relaxed.

4 Most research says you should wash your linen once a fortnight to avoid a build-up of dead skin and sweat, which encourage all sorts of bugs and mites to view your bed as a great home. (This is also another reason never to eat in bed. You'll soon be sharing your food with a bunch of bugs.) Fresh-smelling sheets are such a simple way of making your bed more welcoming.

5 Declutter your room. Tidy up your clothes and keep the laundry basket in the hallway. Clear space (especially floors and surfaces) will lead to a clear mind. No matter how well you think you can cope with mess, it will be affecting you. Losing things, having to jump over stuff and having items that don't belong in your bedroom (like dirty plates and mugs) is stressful and annoying (and quite possibly smelly).

6 This might sound sacrilegious, but get rid of the TV in your room. Don't treat your bedroom as an extension of the living room. Remember, this room is just for sleep and sex.

Make your bedroom a phone-, tablet- and computer-free zone. If you work or surf the net in your bed you'll start associating that room with duty, stress, and stimulation rather than with relaxation and winding down. Finally, if you have pets don't let them into bed with you. Kick Fido out. Their movements can disrupt your sleep.

Your bed

The foundation of a good night's sleep is a comfortable bed, which is why it's worrying that so many people neglect their mattress. You can kind of understand why. They don't advertise being past their sell-by date in the same way other objects do – and shopping for mattresses is never as fun as the people in the adverts make it out to be. However, sleeping on a dust mite laden, allergy inducing sliver of squashy foam isn't good enough – especially if it's over ten years old. A bad bed can steal an hour's sleep a night – and you spend a third of your life in bed – so investing in a good mattress is essential for sleeping (and living) well. It will enhance the duration and soundness of your sleep, support your body and help prevent back pain and joint aches. Think of the benefits.

⑤ Bed buying

It's time to buy a new bed if:

+ You're uncomfortable (this is so obvious, but amazing how often we just ignore it) or if you wake up tired and achy.
+ There are visible signs of wear and tear in your mattress, e.g. sagging, lumps or prominent bed springs.
+ You've turned it over and it's still uncomfortable.
+ You suffer from skin or breathing allergies and have had the mattress for a long time. Disgustingly, dust mite faeces can double the weight of a mattress in ten years – and even the cleanest beds have dust mites.
+ If you feel much more comfortable and sleep better in different beds, i.e. in hotels or at a friend's place.

How to buy a bed:

+ Ask a sales rep for advice. They should know what they're talking about or at least know more than you.

✦ Try before you buy. Go and lie on different mattresses in the showroom, trying out lots of positions to ensure it's right for you. Bounce around. It's the one shop where you're allowed to scramble all over the displays.

✦ If you share your bed with your partner, make sure they're there when you're shopping. You both need to have enough space to be comfortable. If you're very different sizes, think about getting a split mattress (or even pushing two single beds together) so you can both choose the firmness that suits you. Light people tend to need softer mattresses while heavy folk will do better with something firmer.

✦ If you do suffer from allergies do some research online to ensure you steer clear of anything that might set them off, i.e. use foam instead of feathers; make sure the mattress is made out of natural materials to repel dust mites and check it hasn't been sprayed with fire retardant chemicals that could irritate sensitive skin.

Light versus dark

Light triggers a physical reaction in everyone, so a dark room is essential. When it's dark our brains create more melatonin making us feel sleepy. When it's light the reduction in melatonin means we won't feel as tired. We can manipulate light levels to trick our body into thinking it's night when it's day and vice versa – essential for shift workers and people who live in countries where it's either light or dark for most of the day.

Blue light versus red light

Artificial light has different colour wavelengths (bear with us), but most electronic devices (your computer, phone, tablet, etc.) and energy-efficient bulbs emit blue waves – which are exceptionally disruptive at night. Blue light boosts our attention, reaction times and also our mood, which is great for when you want to feel more alert, but terrible for when you want to go to sleep. While any form of light suppresses melatonin secretion, blue light is the biggest culprit. This means alarm clocks and bedside lamps with blue-light emitting bulbs are going to stop you from feeling sleepy and checking phones and computers in bed is guaranteed to wake you up both mentally and physically.

Red waves are the best for recreating the feel of natural light so try to stick to red-wave bulbs wherever possible. Bedside lamps with small low-wattage bulbs are a good bet for creating a soothing pre-sleep mood.

ⓢ Embrace your dark side

✦ Swap conventional light switches for dimmers bought from your local DIY store, and start dimming the lights before bedtime. Bright light inhibits melatonin production, while dim light will trick your brain into thinking the natural light outside is getting darker and so it'll start preparing your body for sleep.

✦ Get an alarm clock with a red light or one that turns off after being set. You can even buy clocks that emit light as if the sun were rising – a gentle and more natural way of waking.

+ Stop looking at bright blue-light emitting electronics (i.e. your computer or phone) at least an hour before bed so your natural melatonin secretion can start.
+ Consider investing in blackout blinds or curtains to make your room totally dark or in the short term buy some black paper or card to stick in the windows.
+ Invest in an eye mask to stop the light interrupting your sleep.
+ Get out during the day or at least open the curtains. The natural light will stimulate the feel-good hormone serotonin, which will make you feel better and less tired. It'll also kick start your circadian timer which means when it gets dark you'll feel naturally sleepy.

Noise nuisance

You can wake up during any of the five stages of sleep (see Chapter 3), but you're more likely to be sensitive to noise in the earlier stages 1 and 2. However, your body is primed to wake you up (whatever stage you're in) if there's a whiff of danger. The ability to be able to keep you and your family safe while asleep is an integral part of being human. As great as that is in theory though, it's not that handy if you've just moved above a twenty-four hour karaoke bar. But don't pull a Van Gogh just yet – there are proactive things you can do to limit noise in your bedroom.

Ⓢ Soundproof your room

As well as literally soundproofing your room's ceiling, floor, and/ or walls (which takes up valuable space and is costly) there are a number of easier ways to get a similar effect:

+ Remove any unnecessary noise. As much as you think you're
  used to that cuckoo clock, it might be contributing to a build-
  up of noise (i.e. a combination of the cuckoo, the watch on your
  bedside table and next door's grandfather clock) so get rid of what
  you can. Also, as Danielle discovered, removing noise from your
  bedroom is a simple way of feeling more in control of your sleeping
  environment.

+ Consider when the heating and hot water turns on and off. If the
  boiler is near your room it might start clattering and clanking in the
  middle of the night.

+ If your partner snores, visit your local chemist to stock up on
  snoring remedies (there are lots of options). Also, if they're lying
  on their back, roll them onto their side – people tend to snore more
  frequently and much louder on their back.

+ Consider buying earplugs. Sounds that you need to hear will still
  get through (i.e. your baby crying or your name being called loudly
  – we're programmed to pick up on those sounds no matter what's
  going on around us) yet non-threatening noises will be muffled.
  However, there is a downside to earplugs: your own bodily sounds
  will be amplified i.e. your breathing and swallowing. If you find this
  is the case try white noise.

+ White noise. You can download apps or buy specific white-noise
  machines that emit a neutral background sound that masks anything
  happening below that level; it's pretty clever. Your inner sensors are
  triggered to pick out any noises that could signal danger – voices,
  crashes and bangs – but you won't hear any unnecessary distractions
  such as low-level conversations, TV or music.

+ Don't sweat the big stuff. If you live next to a high-speed railway you will eventually get used to it and eventually sleep through. Your mind will accept that this is a regular noise and not a danger.

Temperature tests

Sleep much prefers cold temperatures to hot ones. There is no one-temperature-fits-all as far as sleep is concerned, but when you hit sleep stage 2 your core body temperature naturally drops to keep everything ticking over – you don't want to hike it up again by being stuck in a stuffy room.

Ⓢ Turning down the heat

+ If you're cold, get a bigger duvet instead of ramping up the room temperature. A cool room with a duvet thick enough to keep warm is ideal.

+ Invest in a hot-water bottle or bed socks to keep your feet warm. Feet often get colder than the rest of your body and this will save you having to heat the whole room.

+ Change the thickness of your duvet with the seasons – a thinner duvet or sheet in summer and thicker in winter.

+ Wear temperature-appropriate clothing. It may sound obvious, but it's bizarre how often we just stick with what we're used to even if we know it's not working.

+ Open a window if you can to allow fresh air to circulate.

⑤ Your bedroom behaviour sleep diary

After you've made these changes (and you have to tackle every area), start your sleep diary for another week and then assess what has happened. Were there any positive changes in how long you slept for and how soundly? Does your bedroom feel more conducive to sleep? Do you feel calmer when you go into the room? Hopefully the answers to all those questions are yes, because there's no way limiting noise and keeping things dark and tidy will actually disturb your sleep. Also, identify what you think really made a difference (buying an eye mask or moving your TV out of the room, for example). You'll feel more in control and as though you're making progress if you can identify things that have been contributing to the problem.

Thoughts to take away

✓ Adapting your bedroom and creating a calm haven for yourself will make you feel more in control of how well you sleep

✓ Making lots of little changes will all add up to one big positive change

✓ Your bedroom should only be for sleep and sex! Making these changes will reassert those associations

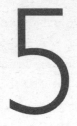

Eats, Sleeps
and Leaves

We can pretty much guarantee that what you're doing (or not doing) during the day will be contributing to your sleeping problems. There are lots of things you can either adopt or sacrifice in your day life that will encourage sound slumber.

Changing life to suit your sleep

It might sound drastic, but if you're serious about addressing your sleeping problems you're going to have to change what you do during your 'day life' to suit your 'night life'. Just like all the tips and tricks for creating a relaxing bedroom, the little things you do day-to-day might not seem important when you look at them individually, but collectively they make a big difference to how well you sleep.

Downing espresso shots and then composing emails in bed until 2a.m. may not bother people without sleeping issues, but unfortunately they'll definitely bother you. Cutting down on some 'bad' habits (bad as far as sleep is concerned) might feel pretty boring to start with, but if it helps you get to sleep it'll be a totally worthwhile sacrifice. And it's not forever – as soon as your sleep is back on track you can start experimenting with re-introducing them into your life.

Sleep's enemies
Caffeine

Caffeine is a stimulant, meaning it will increase your heart rate, produce adrenaline and suppress your melatonin levels. Most people know that caffeine is present in tea and coffee, but it's also in chocolate (yep, sorry) and some medications so you might not even be aware you're ingesting it.

Don't panic, you don't have to cut caffeine out altogether – your morning coffee (or two) isn't a problem at all as it's early in the day – you just have to be aware of it in the evenings as that's when it will disrupt your sleep.

You might find that cutting down could make you feel worse for a while. Caffeine is addictive and headaches are a common symptom of withdrawal. Don't let this put you off though, your body will soon get used to the new status quo and then you'll feel back to your best (especially as your sleep should have improved).

S Don't have caffeine four to six hours before going to bed. Your body takes time to break it down, so it will still be affecting you for hours after you've had it. Try herbal teas or decaffeinated drinks instead.

Nicotine
Nicotine is also a stimulant and highly addictive. It arouses your nervous system and will increase your respiratory rate, your heart rate and your blood pressure – none of which will leave you feeling chilled out and ready to snooze. Research has shown that regular smokers take longer to fall asleep and get less sleep compared to those who have never smoked (approximately fourteen minutes less per night).

S Quitting is pretty much the only way to stop nicotine affecting your sleep, but if you can't, don't want to, or are in the process of trying to give up, there is one thing you can do to make life easier: never light up in the middle of the night. Your body will start expecting this regular nicotine hit and wake you up at silly hours. If you're genuinely ready to give up, visit your GP who can help you form a plan of action and put you in touch with support groups.

Alcohol
While it may seem like a good way to relax and unwind before bed,

alcohol will lead to poorer quality, more fragmented sleep. You might find yourself waking up early or intermittently and be unable to get back to sleep. It's also a diuretic so you'll probably have to get up several times to go to the toilet or drink buckets of water because you feel dehydrated. It can lead to a vicious circle: you're worried about not sleeping so drink alcohol to unwind, sleep poorly and then resort to more alcohol again the next night.

S Try to avoid alcohol at least four to six hours before going to bed so your body can rest instead of digesting. However, if you'd rather risk being up all night than lose the comfort of that evening glass of red, try out different amounts so you can work out your tolerance levels. (This relates directly to the sleep diary strategy at the end of the chapter.)

Non-alcoholic drinks

No doubt you've had it drilled into you for years that drinking gallons of water is good for you – and it is. However, drinking too much of any drink before you go to bed can mean you'll be back and forth to the bathroom all night. A full bladder will wake you up demanding attention.

S If you find you're nearly spending more time in the toilet than in bed, try to redistribute the amount of fluid you drink, taking in more in the morning and then levelling out during the day. Drink nothing two hours before trying to sleep and ensure you go to the toilet before getting into bed.

Sleeping pills

Sleeping pills can be an effective short-term solution to sleeplessness, but on-going use can encourage dependency, interfering with your natural sleeping patterns. They can actually prolong your sleeping issues as you're not fixing the problem of why you can't sleep. Some pills can also make you feel drowsy during the day so you'll start napping – another unwelcome change to your natural sleeping rhythms.

Ⓢ Using sleeping pills long-term isn't great. Always speak to your doctor both before taking pills and when coming off them. Never stop taking medication suddenly.

Napping

Napping causes more problems than it solves. It makes it harder to fall asleep at night and you're more likely to wake up sporadically. Not only are you lessening your drive for sleep (and so interfering with the sleep homeostat), but if you nod off on your sofa you're weakening the important association with your bed and sleep. And, if you nap regularly, you'll be conditioning your body to expect a nap each day, so if for any reason you can't snatch forty winks you'll feel even more tired and sluggish.

Ⓢ Just don't. It's a short-term solution to a long-term problem that will only exacerbate your sleeping problems. It's like jet lag – you have to ride out the tiredness until you can go to bed at a reasonable hour and then you'll be more likely to sleep through the night.

Clock watching

Counting down the hours you have left to sleep – 'I'll get three hours
if I fall asleep now' – is one of the loneliest and most panic-inducing
things you can do. You'll start punishing yourself for not having fallen
asleep yet, leading to anxiety about how you'll cope the next day.
Clock-watching actively keeps you awake as your brain is primed
to assess how long you've been asleep. You'll suddenly jerk awake
thinking, 'Was I asleep?' and then chastise yourself for waking up when
you realise you actually were.

S Turn your clock around and don't look at it. (Doubly helpful if it's
emitting blue light.) Looking isn't going to solve anything, it's only
going to aggravate your anxiety. If you do wake up knowing it's late
(or very early as the case maybe), tell yourself it's 2a.m. Your brain will
accept this hour without panicking because although it's late, you'll
still be able to get a few hours of sleep before having to get up.

Technology overload

We've mentioned how most gadgets emit a blue light that will
physically bother you, but going online at night will also stimulate you
mentally. In today's twenty-four hour society it can be exceptionally
hard to log-off when you have social media updates coming at you
from all corners. However, trying to think up a continual stream of
witty replies on Twitter will only keep you alert when you should be
trying to sleep.

S Switch off at least an hour before going to bed. The world won't end if you don't contribute to virtual discussions and work will definitely survive without you at night (and realising this by testing it out will feel like a big weight has been lifted off your shoulders).

Sleep's heroes

These are the things that sleep wants most. Bring more of these things into your life and you won't even recognise yourself come night time.

Routine

Going to bed and getting up at roughly the same time every day is a simple way of creating a sleep routine. Your body will start to expect sleep at regular hours, strengthening your circadian rhythm. Be firm with yourself about staying out late for the next few weeks. Once you're sleeping better you can be more relaxed, but it's totally worth coming home a tad earlier now if you're tired. You need to be strict on weekends or days off too, allowing yourself only an hour's lie in. The point is to always be in bed when your body wants to sleep, but not to spend hours lying there when it doesn't.

S Don't ignore it when your body gets tired. If you need to go to bed earlier, then do; if you're not tired when you're scheduled to go to bed, then don't. Try not to cancel any plans no matter how shattered you feel or you'll become even more fixated on the issue of sleep, thinking, 'I can't do things like I used to.' Keeping busy will lift your mood.

Exercise

Exercise will make you feel better both mentally and physically. The endorphins that flood your system will make you feel happier and better able to cope with any lack of sleep and its repercussions. It relieves the stresses of the day and helps you to switch off.

Physically, research suggests that cardio exercise (that gets your blood pumping, heart rate up and makes you sweat) can give you a deeper, sounder sleep so you'll spend more time in the restorative stages 3 and 4. It also increases your metabolism so you won't feel as heavy or bloated.

Ⓢ Try brainstorming a list of exercises that you can easily fit into your day and avoid exercising in the late evening. (Exercise increases adrenaline production making it harder to sleep in the short-term so make sure you give your muscles at least an hour to relax.) You could get off the bus a stop early and walk, work out to an exercise DVD first thing in the morning or join a class at the gym.

Food

What you eat will impact on how you sleep and vice versa. The US National Health and Nutrition Survey found that people who slept seven or eight hours a night ate the greatest variety of food, while those who only managed five hours drank less water, imbibed less vitamin C and had less of the trace element selenium (found in nuts, meat and shellfish) which affects thyroid function and can help to maintain a stable metabolism.

Ⓢ A healthy balanced diet will aid sleep, but timing is key too. Try not to eat very late or too much in the evening as your body will still be digesting when you get into bed. However, it's equally important not to go to bed hungry as a rumbling stomach is just as distracting! A light snack an hour before you go to bed can stop a blood sugar drop during the night. (See recommended foods on page 84.)

The ingredients for sleep

The three substances found in food that promote good sleep are:

Trytophan: An amino acid found in all proteins. Tryptophan is used by your body to create serotonin which in turn creates melatonin, 'the sleep hormone'.

Serotonin: The 'happiness hormone' that carries messages between our brain and other cells. It's triggered by sunlight and governs our mood. A lack of serotonin can lead to anxiety, depression and a craving for carbohydrate foods (which commonly contain it). During the night, serotonin is converted into melatonin.

Melatonin: You'll be familiar with melatonin already. It's the hormone that regulates the body's circadian rhythm and promotes restful sleep. This is produced from serotonin and can be found in certain foods. The best way to ensure optimal melatonin production is to sleep in as dark a room as possible. (Avoid taking melatonin supplements as this can adversely affect your body's natural production.)

Ⓢ Five food heroes for sleep

Dairy contains both melatonin and tryptophan, which converts to serotonin. Other dairy products such as cottage cheese, cheese and eggs contain both tryptophan and calcium. (Vegans will need to eat more of other food sources listed).

Carbohydrates stimulate the release of insulin, which clears the bloodstream of amino acids that compete with tryptophan. Complex carbs such as crackers, bread and bagels increase serotonin, while whole grains contain vitamin B, which protects the nervous system and soothes the body and mind thereby combating anxiety, irritability, tension and insomnia. This vitamin group is needed for your body's cells to convert carbohydrates and fats into energy. It is essential for fighting chronic stress and aids the function of a healthy nervous system.

Protein-rich foods such as turkey, chicken, beef and pork contain tryptophan while salmon and herring contain omega-3 fatty acids (DHA) which stimulates melatonin production.

Fruit such as bananas promote both serotonin and melatonin production, but also contain magnesium, a natural muscle relaxant. Cherries are brilliant, full of anti-inflammatory vitamins and melatonin.

Nuts are a great source of melatonin, particularly walnuts. Research found that people's levels of melatonin rose threefold after eating walnuts so grab a handful as an afternoon or evening snack.

Ⓢ Your updated sleep diary

Add some new questions to your sleep diary, this time you will also be monitoring your caffeine, alcohol and nicotine intake and your diet.

Sleep experience (additional questions)	Monday
What was your bedtime snack and what time did you eat it?	
What exercise did you do during the day?	
How many cigarettes did you smoke and when?	
Did you have caffeine and if so, when?	
How many alcoholic drinks did you have and when?	
Did you take sleeping pills?	

When the week you're recording is up, review the diary. Did your sleep improve? What was the hardest change to make? Do you think it was worthwhile?

The more you practise these lifestyle changes, the easier they'll become. Noting things down in the diary will make you aware of what is working and what isn't and will also force you to acknowledge any bad habits. Some things are such an integral part of our lives that we do them on autopilot – eight cups of tea a day will invariably be contributing to your sleeping problems, but you might not have even been aware you drink that much. Filling out the table will force you to confront the things that might be maintaining your sleeping problems and seek ways to tackle them (e.g. try decaffeinated tea).

⑤ Good habit mind map

Fill in a new mind map focusing on the bad habit that you've found hardest to break – perhaps you're trying to stop smoking during the night or have ditched your 8p.m. espresso hit. Write about how sticking to a new regime made you feel emotionally and physically, what you thought and what it made you do or consider doing. We have filled out an example below.

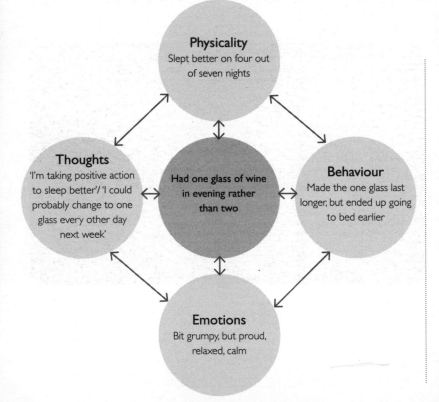

Physicality
Slept better on four out of seven nights

Thoughts
'I'm taking positive action to sleep better'/ 'I could probably change to one glass every other day next week'

Had one glass of wine in evening rather than two

Behaviour
Made the one glass last longer, but ended up going to bed earlier

Emotions
Bit grumpy, but proud, relaxed, calm

Limiting your wine intake alone may not alter how you sleep, but when you add it to a change of diet, cutting down on caffeine, exercising more, and a new sleep routine, your ability to nod off will definitely improve. Don't expect miracles – you're not suddenly going to snooze like Sleeping Beauty. However, you will notice a difference week by week. Your body might take a while to get used to the changes, but it'll soon settle down. You'll find the fact that you're taking proactive steps to improve things is really motivating.

Thoughts to take away

✓ Changing what and when you eat and drink (and go to bed) will massively improve your chances of getting to sleep

✓ Caffeine, nicotine and alcohol are sleep's natural enemies so avoid them while winding down during the evening

✓ Your new day time habits will seem less restrictive when you start experiencing the results!

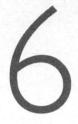

The Rest of
Your Life

Learning to relax is a skill – a really chilled out enjoyable skill – that will change your perspective on sleep. Here's your new snooze-inducing guide to resting and winding down.

Why resting is so important

You have to change how you feel physically in the lead up to going to bed, in order to be in the right frame of mind to sleep. If you're all riled up like a boxer you're not going to pass out unless someone knocks you out.

Relaxation is commonly used as a form of therapy for insomnia. It's impossible to be mentally agitated when you're physically totally relaxed. More than fifty studies over the past thirty years have shown that feeling relaxed produces improvements in how well people rate the quality of their sleep and how quickly it took them to drop off (on average 20–30 minutes quicker). It's amazing how hard it is to rest when you're stressed. If you always dread going to bed your body reacts accordingly – your muscles tense, heart rate rockets and mind races. It recognises the feeling of fear and prepares you to either fight or run away from the threat. It's just trying to protect you, but unfortunately this is the least conducive mental and physical state for falling asleep imaginable.

Example: New mum Niamh's nightmare

Niamh's son, Adam, was six weeks old. He was her first child and she'd been warned about the sleepless nights – but nothing could have prepared her for this. She hadn't slept longer than a few hours a night for the last three weeks.

⋯⋗ At first she'd just wake up whenever he fretted or needed feeding and then drop off again, but she quickly stopped being able to get back to sleep. She knew he'd wake up again in a couple of hours and so felt under huge pressure to snatch what sleep she could. This pressure led to panic and now she couldn't sleep even when Adam was snoozing peacefully. She felt like a mumbling, shuffling corpse. She couldn't empathise with other new mums because she wasn't suffering from a broken night's sleep – she was suffering from no sleep.

She dreaded the evenings as she'd mentally and physically prepare herself for battle; spending hours feeling as tense as a coiled spring. She'd watch her partner and Adam sleeping soundly as the hours ticked by, feeling despair. She knew she wasn't suffering from depression – she felt okay in herself – but she was becoming more lonely and desperate the longer the sleeplessness continued.

Niamh's mind map looked like this:

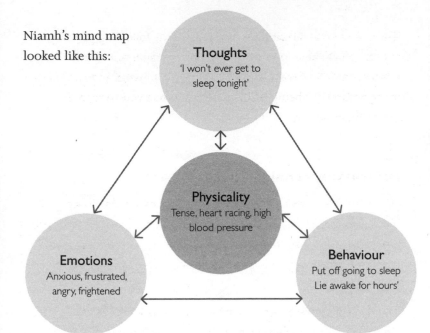

Thoughts
'I won't ever get to sleep tonight'

Physicality
Tense, heart racing, high blood pressure

Emotions
Anxious, frustrated, angry, frightened

Behaviour
Put off going to sleep
Lie awake for hours'

The best possible thing for Niamh to do is to try to relax before getting into bed. Stress and anxiety has made her bed something she's frightened of and her body responds to these feelings just as it would if she were facing an axe-wielding maniac. (And you're never going to nod off if faced with an axe-wielding maniac.)

How to relax

Relaxing deactivates the body's arousal system, which will calm down your thoughts, your body and your emotions. It will also make you less likely to do anything that will discourage sleep – such as avoiding going to bed or starting a new work project at 1a.m.

There are several relaxation techniques on the following pages. You should try all of them to find the one that best suits you. Don't dismiss any as airy-fairy gibberish – they're all proven to work and you might surprise yourself by being really good at the one you were most sceptical about.

Relaxation technique guidelines

✦ Practise at least twice a day for ten minutes each time – once when you're not actually trying to get to sleep so you can really get to grips with the strategy (and also as a handy way of chilling out during the day) and once as part of a wind down routine before you go to bed.

✦ Find a quiet private place where you won't be interrupted or distracted – and turn your phone off. You can't relax if a jaunty ringtone is vibrating in your ear every two minutes.

✦ Get into a comfortable position where your entire body, including your head, is supported i.e. lie on the floor, on a sofa or on a bed. If you can't lie down just sit in a comfy chair. (When lying on the floor you can also slip a pillow beneath your knees for further support.)

✦ Loosen any tight clothing and remove any accessories, e.g. your watch, glasses, jewellery – even your contact lenses. Anything that could move and distract you. ⋯⋰

◆ Give yourself permission to ignore any worries for those ten minutes. This technique should take precedence over everything. Reassure your brain that you can start panicking about life again when the exercise is over – you're just postponing the thoughts, not dismissing them. The success of relaxation depends on your focus and determination to make it work.

◆ Do not try to control your body – just let what happens happen. Free yourself from any worry or judgement about how well you're doing. The whole point of this is to relax. Thinking, 'Well this isn't bloody working,' isn't relaxing. Trust yourself – this will work if you let it.

◆ Consider recording the exercise instructions onto a tape so you can listen as you go along rather than try to remember everything.

◆ And finally – be patient. Relaxing isn't automatic, it's something people with a tendency to feel stressed and anxious have to learn. It will get easier the more you practise.

Ⓢ Deep breathing

Concentrating on your breathing is a brilliant way to focus on the here and now – no matter what's on your mind. It will allow you to slow down both physically and mentally. And the best bit is you can do this five-step exercise anywhere.

1 Rest your hand on your stomach. Inhale slowly and deeply through your nose, keeping your shoulders relaxed. As you inhale push your abdomen out and feel your hand rise.

2 Hold for two seconds.

3 Exhale slowly through your mouth and feel your stomach deflating. As you blow air out, purse your lips slightly, but keep your jaw relaxed. You may hear a soft 'whooshing' sound as you exhale.

4 Smile as you breath out. Smiling actually makes your feel better: think of something or someone you love or just smile for no reason.

5 Repeat for several minutes until you feel calmer.

⑤ Progressive muscle relaxation

Over fifty years ago physician Dr Edmund Jacobson discovered that if you tense a muscle for a few seconds and then release it the muscle will relax completely – much more than it would if you hadn't tensed it.

When stressed your muscles are naturally in a state of tension and can be for some time without you even noticing. Tensing and then consciously releasing various muscle groups throughout the body produces a deep state of relaxation which is proven to relieve many conditions including insomnia. The exercise will also clear your mind as you're being forced to concentrate on your body rather than on day-to-day issues. As soon as worries wander into your head (and they will, it's totally natural), kick them out and bring your mind back to what you're doing.

When you release your tensed muscles it's recommended that you say either out loud or in your head, 'And let go' or 'I'm letting go now'. It may sound ridiculous, but it's very important. It means you're consciously taking control of the exercise – rather than just releasing the muscle, you're choosing to – and it will help you to focus on the feeling of release. By talking yourself through it your mind has no choice but to stay on the exercise. There's no point tensing your arm and then continuing to think about how you won't sleep later on.

The tips below should be employed for every stage of the exercise.

+ When you tense, tense as tightly as possible without straining yourself.
+ Hold the tension for at least ten seconds.
+ When you release say, 'Let go', in your head or out loud.
+ Concentrate on the feeling of tension leaving your muscle as it goes limp.
+ Relax for 15–20 seconds, relishing how good it feels.

Ⓢ Relaxation exercise

+ Take three big 'abdomen' breaths (from the breathing exercise on page 94) and as you exhale imagine all the tension and stress of the day leaving your body.
+ Clench your fists tightly for ten seconds. Concentrate on the feeling of tension and visualise the muscles tensing. Say, 'Let go', and release.
+ Tighten your biceps by drawing your forearms towards your shoulders. Hold, 'let go', and release.
+ Tighten your triceps (the muscles on the undersides of your upper arms) by extending your arms out straight and locking your elbows. Hold, 'let go', and relax.
+ Tense the muscles in your forehead by raising your eyebrows as far as you can. Hold, 'let go', and release. Picture your forehead muscles

becoming smooth as you relax. Focus on your face. Clench your eyelids tightly shut. Hold, 'let go', and release. Tighten your jaw by opening your mouth as wide as possible. Hold, 'let go', and release – letting your lips part and jaw hang loose.

+ Push your head into the pillow it's resting on, tensing the muscles in the back of your neck. (Be very careful to avoid any strain.) Hold, 'let go', then relax. People tend to hold a lot of tension in this area so repeat if necessary. Raise your shoulders up to your ears, and let them drop down again. Push your shoulders as far back as you can. Hold, 'let go', and relax. Repeat if necessary.

+ Suck your stomach in. Hold, 'let go', and release, imagining a wave of relaxation spreading through your abdomen.

+ Arch your lower back towards the ceiling. Hold, say 'Let go', then release. (Omit this stage if you suffer from back pain.) Tense your bum. Hold, 'let go', then relax and imagine tension flowing out from the muscles in your hips.

+ Squeeze your thighs all the way down to your knees, tightening up your hips too. Hold, say 'Let go', and relax. Pull your toes towards the ceiling, tightening up your calf muscles (you can flex to avoid cramping). Hold for a moment and then let go. Curl your toes downward, then release. Mentally scan your body for any residual tension. If a particular area still feels tense, repeat the exercise for that muscle.

+ Picture a wave of relaxation flooding through your body, starting at your head and penetrating every muscle group all the way to your toes.

S Imagery training

This one might take a bit of getting used to. It involves the use of visualisation techniques to focus your attention on peaceful or neutral images, lowering your arousal responses and making you feel calm both mentally and physically. Imagery takes practise so don't try it for the first time before you go to bed or you'll feel anxious when it doesn't work immediately. Instead, practise for ten minutes during the day until you're totally confident and then put it into action during your wind-down routine on page 102.

Go somewhere you won't be disturbed. Sit or lie down.

+ Close your eyes and imagine a place of tranquillity. Somewhere you can feel completely relaxed – perhaps a sunny deserted beach, a lake beside some mountains, your favourite armchair or sitting with your favourite person.
+ To get to this place you have to descend a staircase of ten steps. Picture yourself standing at the top of the staircase, ready to take your first step down. You're calm, relaxed and looking forward to arriving.
+ Imagine yourself sinking softly into each step – as if it's made of warm sand – and feel all the tension you've carried during the day leave you as you count the steps from 10 to 0.
+ As you get to zero, say the word in your head and step into your calm place. Look and move around, noticing the colours, listening to the sounds and imagining the smells and textures.
+ Make the image as vivid as possible, noticing little details: what are you wearing? Do you have bare feet – is sand running through your toes? Incorporate all your favourite things that make you feel safe:

the sound of the sea, the feel of sun on your skin, or the smell of a particular scent.

Once this place and experience is lodged in your memory whenever you feel stressed or anxious you'll be able to summon it and your body will recall the feeling of calm.

⑤ Mindfulness

Mindfulness is different to relaxation — it is a brilliant meditative practice that focuses your brain and body on the present — on what's going on around you rather than what's going on inside your head. It is proven to positively influence your emotions, your nervous system, stress hormones, the immune system and … yes, even sleep.

Mindfulness is all about encouraging yourself to see thoughts as just thoughts and your emotions as just feelings. When it comes to insomnia it neutralises the distress and panic associated with not being able to get to sleep. It's about taking control of your mind rather than letting your mind control you so you're in a better place mentally — and therefore physically — to drop off.

Mindfulness is all about being non-judgemental and accepting. By not judging your ability to sleep and just accepting things as they are you'll feel less tense and therefore put yourself in a better position to sleep. By accepting what's going on you can then choose what to do, i.e. if you can't sleep and don't feel tired, get up and do something else (something relaxing) until you do feel sleepy. Knowing that short consolidated sleep often feels more satisfying than longer fragmented sleep should stop you feeling anxious if you keep waking up.

A pilot study evaluated a six-week version of a mindfulness programme on a sample of thirty participants with insomnia. Half of the participants reported experiencing a 50 per cent or greater reduction in the total time they were awake and all but two participants scored below the cut off for clinical insomnia at the end of treatment.

Ⓢ Mindful about sleep

Practise the exercise shown below during the day, before you go to bed and, if necessary, when you wake up in the night.

1 Imagine yourself on a riverbank, watching the river flow past as the sun shines and sparkles on the water.
2 You notice a large tree over-hanging the river and as you watch a leaf falls and drifts downwards, landing on the water before floating away downstream.
3 Another leaf falls and then another.
4 As the next leaf falls put one of the negative thoughts you have about sleep onto the leaf, without analysing it or assessing it.
5 Place the thought on the leaf and as it hits the river watch it float away.
6 As the next leaf falls do the same – put a thought onto the leaf, watch it land on the water and float away.
7 Feel the water sweeping you towards sleep as your worries are swept away.

This is just an example scenario, feel free to adapt it. The point of this is to get out of your head – to stop stressful thoughts about not sleeping stopping you from sleeping. Instead of getting bogged down in your thoughts, you just acknowledge them and then let them go.

⑤ Your relaxing mind map

After trying out all of the relaxation techniques fill in a mind map focusing on one of the exercises in particular or all of them. How did you feel before and after? Be honest – if you thought, 'this is complete rubbish' about one exercise and felt no different afterwards, write that down.

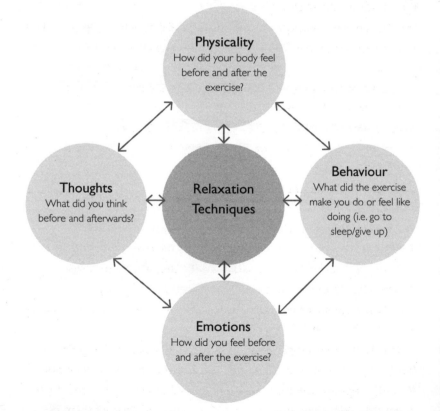

Physicality
How did your body feel before and after the exercise?

Thoughts
What did you think before and afterwards?

Relaxation Techniques

Behaviour
What did the exercise make you do or feel like doing (i.e. go to sleep/give up)

Emotions
How did you feel before and after the exercise?

Was there one relaxation exercise you found particularly helpful? Did it affect your thoughts as much as your body? Did your inhibitions about how you were doing and whether you looked crazy stop you from fully investing yourself in what you were doing? Filling in the mind map should help you see that relaxation affects every part of your sleep experience. However, if you haven't found the exercises as helpful as you'd hoped, it will also flag up where things are going wrong. For example, if you wrote 'this is a load of nonsense' in the 'thought' section then that will have affected your behaviour, your body and your mood.

You can now choose whether you want to have another shot at the exercise while trying to be more open-minded. Just as you can't force yourself to sleep, you can't force yourself to relax. You have to choose to. If you're not a very chilled out person these techniques are going to take some practise. Keep going, the more you do them the quicker your body will shift into feeling relaxed.

Winding down

Creating an evening wind-down routine (of which relaxing or mindfulness will definitely play a part) will make you feel more in control. You'll develop a pattern that your body will recognise and so instinctually start preparing itself for sleep.

Ⓢ Your wind-down routine

Design a one-hour routine that starts before you go to bed. Brainstorm a range of stuff that you enjoy and that de-stresses your mind. Below are some ideas to kick off with:

✦ **Reading.** Whether you're into gore-heavy horrors or bawdy bodice-rippers, reading gives your brain a break from dwelling on worries and stops you trying to multi-task. Be wary of suddenly realising you've read a chapter without taking in a single word though – you can't be absorbed if you're thinking of other things. Also, stop reading in bed. While you're suffering from sleeping problems your bed needs to be for sleep and sex only. Read somewhere else so your body and mind only associate getting under the covers with sleep.

+ **Having a bath.** Baths are a brilliant way to relax. There's something hedonistic about giving yourself time to just chill out. Also, research shows that when you step out of a hot bath your body temperature drops – the same physical response when you sleep – leaving you feeling tired.

+ **Aromatherapy.** Certain essential oils promote relaxation (chamomile, lavender, bergamot, jasmine, rose and sandalwood). Add some drops to your bath and sprinkle it on your pillow.

+ **Massage.** Beg your partner for a quick shoulder or back massage.

+ **Try yoga or meditation.** Grab an instruction manual or DVD and give it a try.

+ **Make a playlist.** Pick tunes that you find relaxing, not stimulating.

+ **Drink warm milk.** Studies have shown warm milk often reminds us of our childhood and tempts us to sleep. However, even if you didn't drink it as a kid, it contains tryptophan which encourages tiredness.

+ **Have a snack.** As mentioned in the last chapter a small snack an hour before going to bed can stimulate tryptophan, serotonin and melatonin production.

+ **Watch TV.** Make sure you watch something that finishes at a reasonable time and be strict with yourself about turning it off when it's over. Don't start watching a thriller at 10p.m. if you're aiming to go bed at 11p.m. You'll stay up as you'll be overly stimulated. (Particularly tough if it's a brilliant box set, but you won't thank yourself for a twelve episode TV marathon in the morning.)

As a general rule avoid doing anything late at night that will stimulate you – like a crisis phone call with your mate (call her earlier) or starting a new work project (start it in the morning). Also, make sure you have completed all your essential chores before you start winding down. There's no point getting to the end of your hour, feeling blissfully relaxed and then mopping all the floors.

Your wind-down routine should include at least one of the relaxation techniques or a mindfulness technique from the start of this chapter. Here's an example:

An hour's wind down (aiming to be in bed by 10.30p.m.)

9:30p.m.	Watch half an hour of a favourite comedy series
10p.m.	Start running a bath
10–10:10p.m.	Dim the lights and practise imagery relaxation technique while the bath's running
10:10p.m.	Sink into a hot bath
10:30p.m.	Take a warm drink (herbal tea or plain old-fashioned milk) to bed

Your routine can include anything you fancy (that's relaxing) and can last for as long as you want. While we recommend an hour we know that won't always be practical. However, while you're trying to sort out your sleeping patterns ensuring you have at least a bit of time for yourself before you go to bed (even if it's not a whole hour) is essential. If you go to the pub every night, come home half an hour early for the next couple of weeks just so you have some time to relax. Or if you have a family to look after, inform them that you'll be taking some time out and you're not to be disturbed Practise your relaxation technique and read a book for fifteen minutes – anything so you are consciously trying to switch off. Taking this time out for you will really change how you feel about sleep.

Thoughts to take away

✓ Learning to relax takes practise, but it will change your life

✓ An official wind-down routine will prepare you mentally and physically for sleep

✓ Being strict about having time to yourself before going to bed will pay off when you're snoring like a professional

7

Banish Your Negative Thoughts

Negative thoughts are to sleep what kryptonite is to Superman – they ruin everything. This chapter shows you how to change how you think about sleep allowing your body and mind the space it needs to rest.

No rest for the worried

We know that most sleep issues are caused by a stressful circumstance, having something important on your mind (that's not necessarily negative), an upsetting life event or a disruption to your sleeping environment. On the whole we expect that when these problems go away our sleeping patterns will revert back to normal. However, when sleep starts playing up, your attention can shift from the original problem and focus on sleep instead – so even when the issue that triggered the problems is fixed, your sleeping issues remain.

Anxious thoughts about sleep can dominate your time and head space, which is frustrating because they're a massive waste of time and they'll actively stop you sleeping.

Sophie's sleep issues

Sophie was in an unhappy relationship and didn't know how to get out of it. Her partner, Richard, was emotionally dependent on her and had made it clear that he wouldn't cope well with her leaving. She hadn't been able to sleep for weeks, lying awake at night anxiously thinking over how, when and if she could do it.

At work Sophie felt sluggish. She'd been late handing a proposal in and had made a couple of mistakes that were totally out of character. All she could focus on were 'what ifs'. 'What if he falls apart if I leave?' 'What if I can't cope at work because I'm not sleeping?' She felt lonely and isolated. Sophie was so tired and overwhelmed ⋯⋮

⋯ she felt as though she couldn't relate to her friends and so started avoiding social occasions. She didn't want to go home though, so spent a lot of time on her own in cafes and pubs.

Sophie thought that if she slept properly she'd be better able to manage what was happening with Richard – so she switched her worries from him to sleep. She started drinking in the evenings and when she went home she'd stay up late watching films. Sophie's sleeping issues became worse and worse until she had to sign off work with exhaustion.

A couple of weeks later it became clear to Sophie and Richard that something had to give. The breakup was as devastating as they'd expected, but they both knew it was the right thing to do. But Sophie still couldn't sleep. Her body clock was all messed up. The fact that taking action in her personal life hadn't solved the sleeping problems exacerbated her emotional fragility. She now spent her nights worrying about whether she would ever sleep normally again – and then those worries triggered thoughts about Richard and whether she'd done the right thing.

When you suffer from poor sleep or insomnia your perspective on life is very different from those who can drop off without a care in the world. You not only worry about sleep, but you'll try to anticipate and control it, make plans around it and make it the focus of your day life as well as your night life. Your negative thoughts cast a gloom over everything – your bedroom, your bed, evenings, mornings, your job, your confidence etc. You'll also chalk up anything else that goes wrong in your life as a consequence of your sleeplessness, i.e. 'this wouldn't have happened if I hadn't been tired' or 'I'd be able to manage this if I could just sleep'.

Over-thinking sleep makes everything worse. You're dwelling on something that you shouldn't have to think about at all, evaluating whether you've slept enough, whether you can cope during the day and trying to guess how you'll sleep in the future. You'll also focus on the symptoms associated with not sleeping, such as fatigue, irritability and low mood. Your body will respond in kind, getting het up and

Increased heart rate, feel tense and alert

Poor sleep

Anxiety

Think, 'I'll never fall asleep tonight and then won't cope tomorrow'

Focus on symptoms i.e. feeling tired and irritable

you inevitably won't sleep, exactly as you feared. However, instead of blaming your thoughts you'll blame sleep – and the whole circle starts again (see previous page).

Remember, you don't think about breathing, you just breathe. You don't think about your heart beating, it just beats. You don't think about swallowing, you just swallow. Sleep should slot neatly into this category because it's something we, as humans, just do. Worrying about it is not only going to make it worse, it's going to provoke negative emotional and physical feelings and unhelpful behaviours.

Your mission is to rediscover your natural sleep rhythms – for sleep to become automatic – which will happen when you put all of our strategies into practise. Once you learn how to stop thinking negatively about sleep and blaming sleep for your problems you'll feel better able to cope with the other things in your life.

Worries and Negative Automatic Thoughts (NATs)

The negative ways you think about sleep can be split into two categories:

1 **Worries:** Consciously dwelling on anxious thoughts. Worries are *deliberate* negative thoughts that you muse on and take your time over. When your worries take the form of 'what ifs' ('What if I don't sleep tomorrow night either?') you're dwelling on something that might never happen.

Worrying about the possibility of something triggers exactly the same response in your body as if it has already happened, your fight or flight response kicks in and you'll actually be less likely to be able to get to sleep. You're actively making what you're scared of happening happen! Worries take up time and have a tendency to spiral so that 'What if I don't sleep tonight?' can quickly turn into, 'What if I fail my exam because I'm exhausted?'

2 **Negative automatic thoughts (NATS):** Thoughts that run through your head without you acknowledging them or even realising they've been and gone.

Unlike worries, NATs aren't deliberate. They are are streams of appraisals and interpretations that run through your head e.g. 'I never sleep properly.' They can be conscious and deliberate, but often they're automatic so you're not even aware of them – you accept them and file them away as statements of fact. They're easy to accept as they can often be plausible (you may not be able to remember the last time you slept 'properly'), but they're always unreasonable and unrealistic (at some point during the last few weeks you will have snatched some sleep or you wouldn't be walking and talking). They're so quick you probably won't even notice them. But just because you don't pick up on them all the time doesn't mean they don't do any damage. They can trigger worries (thoughts you dwell on), make you feel emotionally low and physically tense and also provoke unhelpful behaviour.

If you pick any NAT you have about sleep and challenge it we're willing to bet 99.9 per cent of the time it'll be total drivel and there'll be no proof to back it up. However, this is where your negative biases creep in. When you feel low and run down you need something to blame – sleep – so you'll start looking for proof to defend your gloomy thoughts: 'I messed up that email because I'm tired.' The fact that feeling tired had nothing to do with your mistake won't influence your negatively skewed mind, but it should. You need to change the unhelpful beliefs and attitudes you have about sleep to reduce the emotional distress associated with going to bed. This is the only way that your sleep will return to normal.

The more you believe and accept worries and NATs the worse you're going to feel – and the less likely you're going to be able to get to sleep. Unfortunately, the more anxious you are the more credible, intrusive and harder to dismiss the thoughts become and the more your biases come into play. You have to challenge these thoughts – accept that they're not facts, just hypotheses – and then look for proof against them. For instance, take the email mistake example mentioned above. Instead of immediately blaming the error on being tired you should ask yourself, 'Have I made a mistake like that before when I wasn't tired?' Chances are you have, meaning sleep isn't to blame and your lack of sleep isn't overly influencing your life. Okay, so the bad news is you made a mistake, but the good news is that being tired isn't ruining everything!

Because worries and NATs play an equal role in affecting how you feel about sleep we're sticking them together under a 'negative thoughts' umbrella so we can launch a double assault on them simultaneously.

Your negative thought mind map

Fill in a mind map focusing on a negative thought (either a worry or a NAT) that you've had recently about sleep. Anything that troubles you about getting to sleep, not getting enough sleep, waking up during the night or coping during the day. Then fill in how this thought made you feel emotionally and physically and what it made you do or think about doing.

We have used the email mistake we mentioned above as an example:

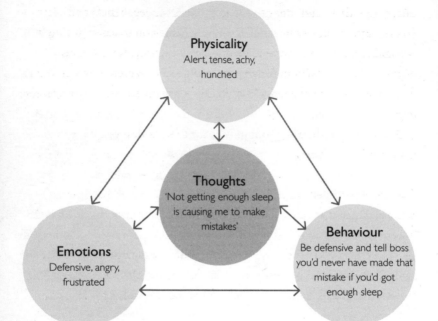

Putting your negative thoughts under a microscope will show you how damaging they are and how they affect every aspect of your life. Yes, sleeplessness is horrible, but worrying about it is a monumental waste of time. If you're not doing anything proactive to improve things, you're actually aggravating the problem.

Coming up with alternatives to negative thoughts will allow you to respond to other thoughts, emotions and physical feelings in more helpful, positive ways, taking the pressure off sleep.

⑤ Becoming a negative thought detective

You need to confront those conniving negative thoughts and interrogate them and identify the negative attitudes, beliefs and biases you're harbouring about sleep. This will enable you to assess if they're rational and if there's any evidence to back them up. Recognising negative thoughts will make you more objective, which is essential for when you come to challenge them and eventually stop them altogether in the next chapter.

Below, we list the key thought biases which both contribute to and maintain sleeplessness.

The fortune teller's error

You anticipate that things will turn out badly and behave as though this is an established fact – 'I'll never sleep tonight'.

⑤ **The truth:** You cannot and do not need to control sleep. You can smooth the process, but sleep is controlled by the sleep homeostat and circadian rhythms. Stop pressuring yourself and let sleep do its job.

The blame game

You blame every problem or issue on the fact that you're not sleeping well – 'I tripped over that step because I'm tired' or 'I argued with my friend because I'm exhausted.'

⑤ **The truth:** Sleep can affect mood, concentration, memory and work performance, but it's not the only cause of these problems. These symptoms can happen for a wide variety of reasons and affect people who do sleep well just as often. Don't use lack of sleep as an excuse for poor behaviour, a lack of effort or just being unlucky.

Catastrophising

You attribute extreme consequences to not falling asleep, overestimating the probability of disaster and underestimating your ability to cope, e.g. 'Everyone thinks I'm rubbish at my job because I'm always tired.'

Ⓢ **The truth:** Sleep debt can be repaid over a period of weeks and months – and even then you only need to repay approximately one-third of what you've lost. If you have a few bad nights' sleep in a row, don't panic – you can make it up. Don't think about it. Knowing this should stop you freaking out about the repercussions on your day life and stop you interfering with sleep by changing your behaviour.

Monochrome thinking

Everything is clear-cut, black and white – 'I had a great night's sleep!' versus 'I had a terrible night's sleep' and 'I feel amazing because I slept well' versus 'I feel hideous because I slept badly.'

Ⓢ **The truth:** There is no magic amount of sleep. A good or bad night's sleep doesn't directly correlate to a good or bad day – you'll have good days when you're tired and bad days when you're not. That's life. Acknowledge that there are shades of grey where sleep is concerned.

Overgeneralisation

You blow up a single negative event, giving it the potential to become a never-ending pattern – 'I'll never sleep again' or 'The next time I get stressed I won't be able to sleep.'

Ⓢ **The truth:** A bad night's sleep doesn't mean a bad week of sleep. Use your sleep diary to compare how you functioned during the day after a particularly bad night – chances are you managed okay. Also, by incorporating all our strategies into your life you will have already seen some positive changes disproving the theory that bad sleep is a never-ending pattern.

Tunnel vision

When you're anxious about sleep, you become biased. You focus on one aspect of bad sleep, ignoring more relevant information. For example, you're convinced your shoulder ache is down to your bad night rather than the game of golf you played the day before.

S **The truth:** Stop your obsession with sleep. Focusing on bodily symptoms will only make them worse and constantly hunting out proof that sleep is ruining your life won't help. Keep busy to distract yourself and focus on the things you can actually influence.

Thoughts to take away

✓ Thinking negatively about sleep will actively stop you sleeping. Calming down your mind will also calm your body, allowing it to rest

✓ Challenging your negative thoughts will prove that things aren't as bad as they seem

✓ Thinking more realistically about sleep will give you a more positive perspective on the rest of your life

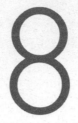

Changing How You Think About Sleep

Now you've identified your worries and NATs about sleep you can confront and test them. This chapter will prove that they're just pointless time-wasters that don't deserve the head space you're giving them and teach you how to get rid of them for good.

How to challenge negative thoughts

Recognising your NATs and worries about sleep will have given you some much needed distance from them. Acknowledging their joint influence on your life is a big step in limiting their power over you. Your negative sleep-based thoughts will be perpetuating the problem. You're now in a position to decide if you want them to continue taking up any time and space in your head. The good news is that they're connected so challenging your NATs will decrease how much you worry about sleep and vice versa. CBT will change any and all dysfunctional beliefs you have about sleep so you won't feel the need to look for the negatives in situations if your thoughts aren't making you feel low and anxious.

Lizzie's long night

Thinking negatively

Lizzie couldn't sleep for the fourth day in a row because she had another stressful day lined up at work tomorrow which she was dreading. It was 1a.m. and she had to get up at 6a.m. She thought, 'I'm not even sleepy yet so I'll never drop off. I'm going to be completely shattered tomorrow and perform badly.' She felt anxious and frustrated, her heart started racing and she felt hot and flustered – making falling asleep even more unlikely.

Challenging the negative thoughts

Even people with insomnia sleep for a bit most nights, but next ·····∵

⋯∴ day they tend to underestimate the amount of sleep they've had. They're expecting to feel tired so they focus on any feelings of exhaustion to back up this view. Believing this puts their body and mind under more pressure which actively stops them sleeping. Lizzie will get some sleep – even if it isn't as much as she needs or wants and she'll be able to catch up with what she's lost, later on. Also, Lizzie might not be at her best the next day, but her body will endeavour to get her through it.

Thinking positively

If Lizzie changed her thoughts to, 'I'm not tired yet, but I usually get some sleep. I'll probably nod off soon if I stop thinking about it,' she'd feel calmer both emotionally and physically and be more likely to fall asleep.

By interpreting your situation more realistically you'll stop putting so much pressure on yourself and instead start taking practical steps towards getting to sleep.

Most of your negative thoughts about sleep are based on misinformation. You might believe that a few bad nights will lead to weeks of the same or that waking up in the night means you'll have a terrible day. These things aren't true, but if you really believe them you'll start making them true. You need to start being more realistic so negative thoughts won't get a foothold and you'll have no need to dwell on fears about the consequences of not getting enough kip.

⑤ Your negative thought diary

Record your negative thoughts about sleep in the diary such as the one opposite. This will make you identify what you're actually worried about (you might think lying awake is your biggest concern when actually it's wondering how you'll feel in the morning) and what is triggering these thoughts. Assessing what kind of thought it is (e.g. the fortune teller's error or catastrophising) will offer up some simple ways of challenging it. Using what you've learned from the book so far and from your sleep diaries you can change your negative gut-reactions to sleep to something far calmer, neutral and less damaging.

Questions to confront your negative thoughts with:

+ What is the evidence for this idea?
+ What is the evidence against it?
+ Why do you think it is true?
+ What are the chances it will happen?
+ What is the worst that could happen?
+ Could you live through it?
+ Is there a more realistic outcome than the one you fear?

By challenging your NATs and worries you're thinking through your options and being proactive. Filling in a diary such as this should convince you that accepting negative thoughts as facts is ridiculous. They're not helping you sleep, they're actually scuppering any chance you have of dozing off.

Trigger	Thought	Type of thinking bias	Challenge to thought	Positive behaviour
Waking up during the night	'I'm not going to be able to cope tomorrow'	The fortune teller's error: I'm anticipating things will turn out badly and acting as if this is a fact	Yes, losing sleep can affect me mentally, but my body will do everything in its power to cope	Don't cancel plans or tell people I feel exhausted. Giving sleep priority in my thoughts will distract me from other tasks
Tossing and turning	'My sleeplessness is making me ill'	Tunnel vision: I'm focusing on one bad aspect of sleep and ignoring more important information	My sleeplessness might be a symptom of my illness rather than the cause	Try to solve both the health issue (visit my GP) and my sleeplessness (employ this book's techniques)
Not getting to sleep	'I've had the worst night's sleep ever last night'	Monochrome thinking: everything is clear cut, black and white	Did I really have my worst night's sleep ever? I can check by looking through my sleep diaries	If I did have my worst night I can see what I did differently, employ all the strategies and check if my sleep improves over a month. If I didn't I should stop making generalisations with no basis in fact
Feeling irritable and arguing with partner	'I'm only arguing with him because I haven't slept well'	The blame game: I'm blaming my problems on a lack of sleep	Irritability is a normal human emotion that also affects people who sleep well. While sleep can exacerbate it, it's not the only cause. I can choose not to be argumentative	Identify the root cause of my irritibility and try to find a way to solve it. If it genuinely is sleep then practise a relaxation technique to calm down

⑤ Reality check

How you feel or think about a situation is not always a good indicator of how things really are. For example, you may be worried that you're slacking at work because you're so tired, yet everyone else thinks you're doing a great job. When you feel negative, worried and run down you're programmed to expect and assume the worst – historically this response is meant to help you sniff out danger, but mostly it just makes you feel bloody awful.

Negative thoughts tend to be very convincing buggers so you need to tell yourself (firmly) that thinking more realistically about situations is the right way to think. The only way to do that is to find proof that both backs up your new more positive thoughts and undermines your negative ones.

Fill out a reality check table (see the example opposite) to test your assumptions and predictions for validity.

Five questions to ask yourself:

1 **Situation:** Write down a specific negative thought in the situation box, e.g.:

   I'm not getting the eight hours' sleep I need a night.

   How I feel when I wake up in the morning determines how I will feel for the rest of the day.

   Everyone knows when I've slept badly.

2 **Prediction:** Next, note down what you predict will happen and how likely you believe it is to happen on a scale of 0–100 (0 = not at all, 100 = totally convinced). You also need to think about how you'll judge whether your prediction was correct or not.

3 **Experiment:** Devise and conduct an experiment to test the prediction.

Situation	If I feel tired I won't have enough energy to see people	I'm not getting the eight hours' sleep I need a night
Prediction + What do you think will happen? + Is it likely? (0–100)? + How will you know if it has?	+ I won't have a good time + I (100) + I'll be bad company and feel irritable	+ I won't cope the next day + I (100) + I won't be able to concentrate so I'll make mistakes
Experiment + How can you test the prediction?	Stick to any plans I have in the diary for the next week no matter how little sleep I get and see if I enjoy myself	Monitor how I get on the next time I get less than eight hours' sleep. Also, be realistic about whether any mistakes I make actually are the result of being tired
Outcome + What actually happened?	I went out on three occasions and actually had a good time. People said they were pleased to see me so I wasn't bad company and I was less irritable than when I was at home worrying about sleep!	I felt tired, but I coped and didn't make any mistakes as a result of sleeping badly. I could concentrate, though some tasks took me a bit longer, but this happens at work even when I'm not tired!
Conclusion + How do you feel about the situation and your prediction after the test? + How likely does your original prediction seem now (0–100)?	The body is designed to handle a certain about of sleeplessness so it's important to keep my worries about sleep in proportion and to stick to my plans as I usually end up feeling better after I've been out + I (50)	On the whole I cope okay after a bad night's sleep. When I feel bad during the night and first thing in the morning I mistakenly assume that I won't manage, but there's a difference between how I feel and what actually happens + I (60)

4 **Outcome:** Review it and write down the actual outcome.
5 **Conclusion:** Jot down how this test made you feel about the initial
   thought. Also, reassess from your new perspective how likely you
   think your original prediction is now, on the same scale (0–100).
   Hopefully the discrepancy between these two figures will convince
   you that you can't predict the future and trying to is making you
   feel stressed for no reason.

Testing your thoughts out will really hammer home how dwelling on
negatives is a waste of time – valuable time that could be spent doing,
well, anything else.

There's no time limit to this exercise – whenever you feel anxious
about the repercussions of getting no sleep, you should test out your
fears using this list of questions. It will reassure you that just because
you're scared something might happen doesn't mean it will. Often
when we're feeling low we actively provoke bad outcomes by behaving
in negative ways. We underestimate our own abilities – and sometimes
it's just easier to blame everything on being tired as it means we don't
have to take responsibility for our actions. Taking proactive steps to
prove ominous thoughts wrong will make you feel better mentally and
physically. Past behaviour is the best predicator of future behaviour –
so if you've coped after a bad night's sleep before then you can again.
Worrying will just maintain your problems, not solve them.

Ⓢ Give up on sleep

You know that 'never give up' team-building T-shirt c.2001 that you
still wear to bed? Well, bin it. By now you're probably bored with us

twittering on about how you can't force sleep, but it's the basis of all your sleeping problems. The only way to deal with this is to stop putting any effort into the physical act of sleeping, which will stop your body from suffering from performance anxiety. To do this you need to trick yourself into believing you don't care about whether you sleep or not. Yes, it's a paradox, which is why this strategy's official – and fancy – title is 'Paradoxical Intention Therapy'. It's recommended by the American Academy of Sleep Medicine and studies show it works by basically getting rid of your preoccupation with sleep. You need to start thinking about those extra hours you spend lying awake as a good thing – time to relax and chill out. Tell yourself you'll fall asleep when you're ready so you don't need to try making your body and mind more susceptible to sleep. You have to stop caring so much.

Yep, this is basically the antithesis to everything you've ever thought or believed is the right way of going about things, but as far as sleep is concerned, not caring is the best thing to do. Stop putting yourself under pressure and you will fall asleep.

Ⓢ Your 'I don't care about sleep' mantras

Come up with a list of statements to reassure yourself that not sleeping isn't the end of the world (because it's not – no matter how much your NATs and worries try to tell you differently). Write them into your notebook so you can have a look whenever you find yourself feeling anxious about sleep. Below are some ideas to get you started:

✦ I can function just fine on little sleep
✦ I always fall asleep eventually

✦ How I feel in the morning won't dictate my day
✦ Small bursts of consolidated sleep can be better for you than long periods of interrupted sleep
✦ I only need to repay one-third of any sleep I miss and can pay it back over a period of months
✦ My body is designed to handle some sleeplessness
✦ I need to be realistic about sleeping and not get carried away by worry

⑤ Thought blocking

Thinking about two things at once really is hard to do, (contrary to what some jobsworths like to preach) – which is where thought blocking comes in. If worries won't go away and leave you alone, then repeat a word that has absolutely no emotional connotations (such as 'the' or 'one') over and over in your head slowly every two seconds with your eyes closed. Keep at it for three to five minutes until your worries have retreated to a dusty corner of your brain. It's just like when you're trying to focus on something while a friend is blathering about something else in your ear – as soon as you tune back into what they're saying you forget whatever it was you were thinking about. By concentrating on your chosen word you'll feel calmer and as though you're wrestling back control of your mind.

This exercise is very similar to counting sheep. The whole philosophy behind counting sheep when you're trying to sleep is to block out any other thoughts that might be agitating your mind. If sheep work for you, go for it!

Thoughts to take away

✓ Worrying will actively stop you falling asleep

✓ Challenging your NATs will prove that sleep isn't the be all and end all in your life

✓ Stop trying to fall asleep and you will!

9

Putting Stress to Bed

We've looked at how to manage worries and negative thoughts concerned with sleep, but dealing with stress about other issues is just as important. Here you'll learn to cope with day-to-day anxieties which will stop them affecting your sleep.

Stress management

Dealing with stress is a normal part of everyday life. We're constantly put under pressure within our roles as friends, relatives, partners, parents, colleagues, neighbours, students, etc. We not only have to live according to our own measures of success, but those of society as a whole. Often the scale of what we're expected to achieve and how we're expected to act can feel frightening, leading us to question our ability to cope.

We live in a twenty-four-hour society where we're expected to be on call non-stop round the clock. We've never been so accessible – if we're not emailing we're tweeting, updating our Facebook status or uploading a picture to Instagram. It can become overwhelming – you're trying to send an email on your iPad, talk to someone on the phone and listen to the news, all while jogging down the street late for an appointment. We're connected to the wider world wherever we are – there's no escape – and it's changed how we go about our day-to-day lives. You don't just watch a TV show anymore, you read an online review about it first and then you tweet what you think about all the characters while you're watching.

Chances are your phone is the last thing you check before you go to bed and the first thing you look at through your sleepy morning eyes. And many of us are working longer and harder than ever before, trying to safeguard our jobs and our futures. We're constantly stimulated and have to multi-task from the second we wake up, which makes it near enough impossible to find any work/ life balance – additionally, those around us have increasing expectations of how accessible we should be.

All of which means you don't even need to be dealing with a

specific issue for worries and anxieties to keep you up at night – just the general onslaught of information you have to process each day will be whipping around your mind like a tornado. Having a wind-down routine is all very well, but if you get into bed feeling mellow and then immediately start planning what you have to do tomorrow, you'll wind up your mind and body again making it impossible to sleep.

Example: David: a life on screen

David worked in advertising, which meant that having and maintaining an online presence was essential to his job – and he enjoyed it. He found discussing stuff and getting feedback from strangers really interesting and sometimes it also served as welcome validation for what he was doing and his ideas.

He spent all day staring at a computer and then would go home and spend the evening staring at his tablet or phone. If someone had told him that he spent upwards of ten hours a day looking at screens he would have been shocked – but it was true. He was addicted to the pieces of plastic in his hand and his online life – he couldn't switch off, even at night. He'd wake up wondering if anyone had replied to his latest status update and if they had, he'd reply straight away. His sleeping patterns were shot to hell, but the thought of neglecting this part of his life sent him into a panic. It took his mind off things and, as he kept telling himself, he had a professional duty to keep it up, even if his social life was pretty much non-existent.

⋯⋮⋯ Then David's bag was stolen on his commute home, complete with his phone and tablet. He was not only furious about the theft, but felt utterly lost. What if someone was trying to call him urgently? What if his Spanish client emailed him back and he couldn't reply? What if someone retweeted his last joke or asked him a question?

David's mind map looks like the one opposite.

It can seem impossible to switch off when you're juggling so many responsibilities, but often we're suffering under an illusion of our own making. Taking David's situation as an example: after his bag was stolen he spent a night feeling cut adrift, restless and even frightened of the consequences – both professional and social – of not having online access. In the morning he got up early, had breakfast and rushed into his office. He logged on and discovered that … nothing – at all – had happened. The email he was sweating about hadn't arrived, the comments on Twitter he'd missed were completely mundane and no one had demanded anything from him. His own internal rule book dictated that he should be accessible 24/7, but externally that need didn't actually exist. Realising this lifted a huge weight off his shoulders. He didn't have to multi-task and run around like a headless chicken all the time. He'd set his own frenetic pace so he could also slow it down – and in doing so he'd make his head and body more amenable to sleep.

On the next pages are some tried and tested ways of limiting the effect stress has on your sleep.

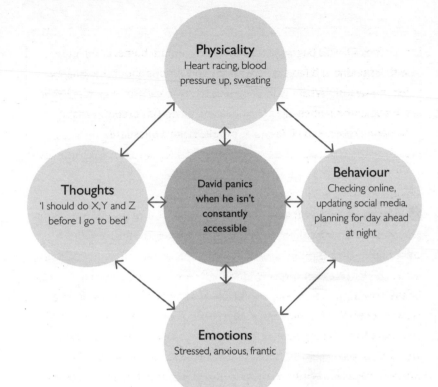

Your 'switch off' checklist

One of the most common symptoms of bad sleep is the inability to 'switch off'. Often when you're busy during the day at work you don't have time to think about life admin such as bills, shopping, DIY, holidays, doctor's appointments or getting your dodgy tooth fixed. All of this takes a back seat and then comes crashing into your head as soon as you crawl into bed. You'll also feel the need to analyse your day and go through what you have to do tomorrow. These thoughts can make you feel physically keyed up and emotionally low, frustrated or anxious. You'll hunt out problems and try to solve them and all the while sleep is shuffling ever further away from the bedroom.

To stop this you need to put up boundaries and maintain them. Learning a few simple stress management strategies is an easy way to switch off so your wind-down routine isn't for nothing.

S Social media blackout

Take note of how long you spend online. It's very easy to reach for your phone on autopilot because you're bored. Stop. Give yourself social media blackout times when you're not allowed to check for any non-essential updates (and no, Hilarious Harry's comments on your favourite TV show are not essential). You'll probably be surprised by how often you reach for your phone without even thinking about it. When you're considering what you want to say and what impression you want to give people your body and mind will feel under pressure. An hour off in the mornings and a few hours in the evenings (on top of your wind-down routine) will give your mind some much-needed time off. Physically remove your phone from hand's reach – try putting it in a different room to help you forget about it for a while.

S Time to reflect

Just as your body gets stuck in certain routines, so does your mind. If you've always thought about and assessed your day while in bed, you'll automatically start to do it as soon as you lie down. To stop this pattern you need to give yourself time to reflect before you're lying in bed. Processing what happened, how you felt and what you thought about it is very important. It offers perspective on a situation, a broader view and some clarity. You're basically tidying up your brain and giving yourself a chance to solve problems and move forward. By building space for this into your day rather than during your sleep time at night you're going to be more focused, less tired and won't allow it to interrupt your sleep patterns.

Set aside fifteen minutes each day (towards the evening or at the start of your new bedtime routine – before you start your wind-down routine) when you can concentrate on thinking about the things you'd normally go over at night. Write yourself a to-do list and prioritise the tasks in order of importance. Ensure you tick things off as you complete them to make you feel motivated. Also, note down three things that you've already completed or that happened and how you felt about them. Schedule the fifteen-minute slot in your diary or on your phone so it's 'official' and you'll be more likely to stick to it.

Seeing things written down will give you a distance from them and enable you to sort through them analytically rather than emotionally. Rather than avoiding thinking about difficulties you're being constructive and this will make you feel calmer and less stressed.

Minimising stress

Stress, anxiety and worry enjoy skipping hand in hand through your mind leaving a trail of chaos in their wake. If you feel under pressure, the fear of what might happen and worries about how you'll cope can keep you up for hours.

Thinking space: Saving time in the long run

You might feel you're too busy to take fifteen minutes out of every day just to think about stuff, but you're no doubt wasting loads more than that worrying and fretting anyway. Scheduling in a consolidated slot just for thinking and assessing your day will not only save you time in the long run, it'll save you a lot of needless stress. Also, it's important to realise that the world won't end if you take a few moments for yourself – and acknowledging that fact will take some pressure off.

Below are some strategies for dealing with different types of stress:

Ⓢ Problem solving and 'worry time'

We've already dealt with sleep-related worries, so the worries we're thinking about here are life-related ones. 'What ifs' about work, money, friends, family and health that might be keeping you up at night and that are usually related to a specific problem or issue.

To deal with these set aside fifteen minutes of 'worry time' (yep, another time slot) during the day when you can sort through them just like you did with the 'time to reflect' thinking-space strategy above. As with that strategy, if there's a sceptical voice in your head whispering, 'Taking another fifteen minutes out of your day – are you crazy?' Shoot it a withering look and ignore it. Step back from the situation for a second and consider how insane it is that you'd consider not doing something that would positively affect your life, all because you can't take a little time for yourself. After you've realised how nonsensical that is you can get started on the task we've got for you.

+ Find a quiet place where you won't be disturbed and write a list of your biggest worries, i.e. 'What if I can't pay my bills this month?' or 'What if I get made redundant?'

+ Ask yourself, 'Is this worry realistic?' if the answer is 'no' then cross it off your list. Why waste valuable time worrying about something that won't happen? However, if the answer is 'yes' then move onto the next step ...

+ What can you do about it? For example, if you're worried you might not be able to pay your bills this month could you call the company to request a payment plan? Could you make yourself a budget so you know exactly what money you have coming in and out? Could you call your bank and ask their advice? Could you ask a family member for a loan?

+ Pick the best idea or one you feel most confident trying out and break it down into smaller more specific steps, e.g. 'Call company at 9a.m. Ask about payment options. Then go through finances – all incomings and outgoings. Work out how much I will have in my account at the end of the month.' Seeing it written down like this will make confronting the issue less intimidating. Allocating a specific time for when you're going to do it will encourage you to start, rather than putting it off for another day.

+ Next, note down any obstacles that might stop you from putting this idea into practise, for example, 'What if the company doesn't have a payment plan?', then work around it. Is there anything you can skip this month to enable you to pay the bill? Could you tie in one of your other ideas and extend your overdraft or ask a family member for a short-term loan?

✦ After your fifteen minutes are up, go back to what you were doing and don't think about the worry again. You have to be strict with yourself about keeping to your schedule and postponing worrying thoughts until the allotted time. You've got a plan now and you're going to put it into action so dwelling on 'what ifs' isn't going to help. If you get into bed and start thinking about it, remind yourself that you can add to or adapt your idea during your next 'worry time' slot.

✦ If you think of any ideas that could help during the day, don't dismiss them, write them in your notebook ready for your next fifteen minutes. After you've noted them down switch your focus back to what you're meant to be doing.

Just the process of writing down problem-solving ideas will reduce their intensity and help you to feel that things are under control. You'll probably also find that often you don't even need the 'worry time' when it arrives as delaying thinking about small concerns can make them redundant because whatever you were fretting about has been resolved by then.

⑤ This is NOT the time

Establish a firm rule with yourself that the next time negative thoughts dance through your head when you're in bed you'll tell yourself, 'This is not the time.' Your bed is for sleeping, not worrying. Just as you now have an allotted time for worrying, when you're in bed that's your allotted time for sleeping – and the times shouldn't overlap.

Whenever you catch yourself stressing or worrying throughout the day, tell yourself you'll come back to the worry at the specified time and then immediately focus your mind back onto the current task. Be strict with yourself on postponing these thoughts – don't let your mind wander into these now time-limited zones. It's become a habit to go over and over the things that are stressing you out, so by postponing them you can build a new, more healthy habit.

Thoughts to take away

✓ Confronting worries and stress about your day life will stop them interfering with your night life

✓ Be strict with yourself about your day and night boundaries – restrict dealing with worries and stress to a specific time during the day

✓ Being proactive about managing stress will automatically decrease how stressed you feel

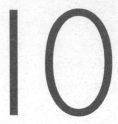

Sleep: The Final Frontier

You've made some steps in the right direction, but now we need to make the association with your bed and sleep concrete and absolutely foolproof. That means shaking up your sleeping routines (possibly quite dramatically). To do that we're sending your body clock to bootcamp. Prepare yourself …

Room for manoeuvre

Now you're a sleep-diary expert whose negative thoughts about snoozing are fading into insignificance we're confident you can handle the next part of the master plan. The activities in this chapter will strengthen the link between your bedroom, bed and sleep. It's all about how you think about your sleeping environment so you need to have worked through the previous two chapters before tackling it. If you suffer from severe sleeping problems then this is the most important chapter for you. These techniques have been used for over thirty years and when it comes to beating insomnia these components of CBT are the most effective.

In Chapter 4 you dealt with some fundamental issues that were detrimental to how you experienced your bedroom and your bed physically (e.g. noise, excess light, comfort, etc.). This should have reconnected you to where you sleep, but there's still more to be done. Some of what we recommend here might raise a few eyebrows, but for people with insomnia this is a crucial part of the process. However, if you'd rate your sleeping issues as mild and what you've put into practise thus far is really working for you, keep on with what you're doing. Only start what we've outlined below if you feel you really need to – this is an advanced stage of therapy and should only be undertaken if necessary.

How you feel about your bedroom and your bed is determined by your experiences surrounding them. If you're a great sleeper you'll associate them with sleep – so when you enter your bedroom you'll think of sleep and even start feeling sleepy. It's the same with any other room that you're familiar with. Walk into your kitchen and you'll think of food or drink and wonder whether you're hungry or want to make a coffee. Wander into your study and you'll think of all the work you have to do. Saunter into your living room and you'll wonder if there's anything good to watch on the TV. When you sleep badly, you'll associate your bedroom with negativity, stress and lying awake. Your bed will conjure up all sorts of negative connotations, e.g. tiredness, frustration, irritation, loneliness.

In order to get to sleep you need to change these negative associations. If you've got this far and things haven't progressed enough for you it's time to take drastic action.

The not-so small print

Be aware that when you first start this strategy you will feel even more tired than before, so be careful when driving or operating heavy machinery. And, if you have a dangerous job or one which involves caring for other people, sleep restriction is best avoided. This is a difficult strategy so if you have any concerns please make sure you speak to your GP first. Having the support of a specialist could be helpful.

⑤ Sleep restriction

This sounds scary and, well, it kind of is – it's by far the most challenging strategy in this book, but it works. Sleep restriction is an intervention process for when your sleep pattern has been out of whack for a long time. It's for people who suffer from severe insomnia and although you may be more tired at first, it'll increase your drive for sleep and give your body clock a much needed kicking. This strategy is only necessary if you sleep less than 85 per cent of the time you are in bed.

You're going to start on a programme of mild sleep deprivation. Yep – seriously. You're only going to be in bed when you're asleep, so no more tossing and turning or dwelling on hideous thoughts under the covers. The whole point of this is to encourage you to fall sleep as soon as your head hits the pillow. Something that might seem a million miles away from what you're experiencing now. This strategy will reset your sleep timer so that you ultimately fall asleep faster, wake up less and achieve better-quality sleep. By limiting the time you're actually in bed your body will conk out as soon as it's allowed to and then you'll hopefully sleep through the night. It'll stop any anticipatory anxiety about the prospect of trying to sleep and what the night might bring and you'll also feel good that you're doing something definitive to address your sleep problems. Your bed will become something wonderful, rather than wicked. Don't worry, there's a method to the madness.

Sleep-restriction rules

These five rules are absolutely essential to the success of a sleep-restriction programme. The strategy won't work if you let any of them slip. ⋯⋰

1 Bed is for sleeping and sex only

No watching TV, using your computer, eating, working, paying bills or even reading while in bed.

2 Have a routine

Set your alarm to sound at the same time each morning. You can allow yourself an additional hour lie-in on the weekend, but that's it.

3 You can't nap – at all

If you're napping during the day, not only are you lessening your drive for sleep and confusing your body about when it should expect sleep, but depending on where you drop off you're also weakening your bed–sleep association.

4 Only go to bed when you feel sleepy

If you're not tired then don't go to bed. Lying in bed feeling frustrated because you can't sleep will just aggravate the problem. You need to become more aware of your body's internal sleep cues. Be alert to when you actually feel tired.

5 If you can't sleep get out of bed

This is tough, but an absolutely essential part of sleep restriction. If you can't fall asleep when you get into bed or can't get back to sleep after waking up, then get out of bed and do something else. If you've been lying awake for roughly fifteen minutes drag yourself out of bed and leave your room. (Don't clock-watch though. Use ⋯⋮⋗

> ·····⁑ fifteen minutes as a rough guide, it doesn't matter if you've been lying there for a little longer or a little less). It may sound hideous, but it's an extremely effective way of maintaining a link between your bed and sleep. Plan what you're going to do when you get up so you're more likely to actually do it. For example, have a book ready to read in the living room. Don't turn on a bright light in whatever room you go into as that will stop melatonin production. Just sit in dim light and try to relax – and then return to bed when you feel tired.

It may seem illogical to cut down the amount of hours you can sleep, but the philosophy is that your body will be so eager to squeeze in as much sleep as it can within the restricted time that you'll nod off straight away. You're merging all the time you normally spend asleep into one clump rather than taking an hour here or there during the night. By not allowing your body to have the luxury of staying awake, you're forcing it to cram in the sleep it needs when it can and resetting your body clock so that sleep becomes more automatic again. When you eventually extend the time you're in bed, your body will have learned to fall sleep immediately and through the night. It'll be a shock, but, quite frankly, your body needs a good shock.

1 To start you need to know how much sleep you're currently getting. Using your sleep diaries work out the average amount of time you spend sleeping per night based on at least ten nights (so, the total amount of hours divided by ten). Also work out what percentage of

the night you were asleep for (total time asleep divided by total time in bed multiplied by 100).

✦ Please note that sleep restriction is only for people who are sleeping for less than 85 per cent of the night and that the restriction should be no less than 4.5 hours. If you are sleeping less than 4.5 hours a night then ignore that figure and use 4.5 as your minimum.

2 Next, set a time to go to bed and a time to wake up based on your average amount of time asleep. So, say you get six hours' sleep on average a night. Keep your established wake-up time and work backwards, i.e. if your alarm is normally set for 7a.m., you should be going to bed at 1a.m. every night. This leaves a six-hour window for you to sleep. You do not have to go to bed at this time if you do not feel sleepy, but this is the absolute earliest you can go to bed no matter how tired you feel. And remember you have to follow the five Sleep-Restriction Rules: if you're not sleepy don't go to bed and if you wake up in the night and haven't fallen back asleep within fifteen minutes, get up and do something else.

3 Aim to extend your wind-down routine so it's preferably over an hour long and make sure you start it in plenty of time before your new bedtime.

4 Keep your sleep diary throughout the task and at the end of each week work out the percentage of time you spent asleep (i.e. total time asleep divided by total time in bed x 100).

5 Once the percentage hits 90 per cent or more, you can increase the amount of time you're in bed by fifteen minutes per week. (So for six hours, you would need to be sleeping for at least five hours and twenty-four minutes for a full week before you could add fifteen minutes.) After you've added this time if you manage to sleep for 90 per cent of the time for the next seven nights you can add another fifteen minutes and so on, week by week. (Don't be tempted to adjust your allowance by more than fifteen minutes as you'll mess up the pattern you've been forming.) If you keep at it steadily like this at some point you'll reach a plateau – the amount of sleep you actually *need*.

This process will be hard physically and mentally, but it'll alter how you sleep forever. You'll be more tired so will sleep as soon as you get into bed and you'll stay asleep throughout the night. And you will manage to cope with your day life reasonably – your body will see to it. Whereas before you might have been in bed for nine hours, but only slept for six (67 per cent of the night), now you'll be sleeping for the majority of time you're in bed – approximately 90–100 per cent.

Yes, this is hardcore, but it works. This will give you the means to work out how much sleep you actually need rather than how much you want and your mind will connect your bed with sleep, rather than with worry and angst. Also, remember when you start that you're just giving your body what it was getting anyway. By the time you're sleeping through you'll be getting the same amount of hours you normally got – but now you're giving yourself the opportunity of extending them long-term.

You might be wary of starting something so consuming and dramatic-sounding – we're not surprised. However, you should note down a list of pros and cons before writing it off. Try adding your own ideas to these:

Pros
+ My sleep will become more automatic
+ I will sleep through the night without waking up
+ I will fall asleep as soon as I go to bed and not lay awake panicking
+ I will stop worrying about sleep because I have a plan
+ I will spend less time in bed feeling lonely
+ I won't dread going to bed, I'll actually look forward to it
+ Short-term pain for long-term gain
+ Insomnia is tough to overcome, but this is proven to work

Cons
+ I'll feel more exhausted at the start
+ It'll be tough to keep to this plan on the weekends

The pros massively outweigh the cons here, and the cons are navigable. You'll only feel more tired for a couple of days while your body adjusts to its new routine and yes, it'll be tough on the weekends, but you can work around that by making morning plans (i.e. go for a walk, pick up breakfast from a local shop, read a book in a cafe with an early-morning coffee) so you don't feel despondent or bored when you have to wake up early and you'll be less tempted to break the rules by sleeping in.

Use the pros to stay motivated and use both the tables in Chapter 8 to challenge any negative thoughts you might be having. If you don't manage to keep to the plan one night, don't worry, just re-read why you're doing it and put it back into action the next night.

Also, make sure you discuss the plan with those living with you as their support will be invaluable once you're in the midst of the routine.

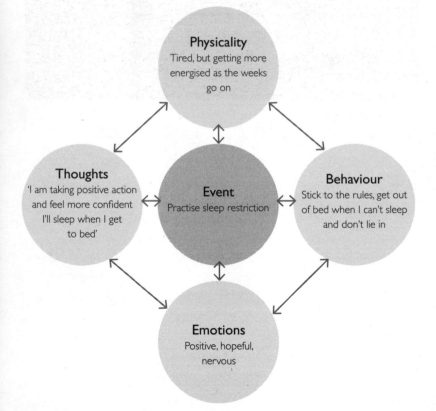

Physicality
Tired, but getting more energised as the weeks go on

Thoughts
'I am taking positive action and feel more confident I'll sleep when I get to bed'

Event
Practise sleep restriction

Behaviour
Stick to the rules, get out of bed when I can't sleep and don't lie in

Emotions
Positive, hopeful, nervous

Thoughts to take away

✓ Only going to bed when you're tired will stop unnecessary angst

✓ You'll start associating your bedroom and your bed with sleep both mentally and physically

✓ Sleep restriction is all about short-term pain for long-term gain

A final message

Congratulations! You've reached the final chapter hopefully feeling far more rested than you did when you first picked up this book.

We're crossing all our fingers that you're well on your way to having and maintaining good sleeping patterns and that your sleep homeostat and your body clock are working together to ensure you're getting the sleep you need.

The fact that you've taken action and chosen not to accept sleep-lessness as a permanent feature of your life is something to be proud of. As you'll now know, you can't control sleep, but you can control how you react to it. If things really have got better then take a few moments to pat yourself on the back, get someone else to pat you on the back or swig some celebratory fizz. Making the changes we recommend will have been – and will continue to be – tough and rewarding yourself for what you've achieved is important, acting as motivation to continue with what you've learned (and if that reward happens to take the form of an all-inclusive holiday then who are we to argue?).

As a means to measure how far you've come please answer the following questions:

1 After reading the book – how do you feel about sleep?

   A The same – no change

   B A smidgen better – starting to think this all through

   C Better – putting in place improvements

   D Amazing – transformed

If you answered option A did you really invest all your energy into the strategies? Are you willing to try them again? If you are still having difficulties and the book hasn't helped you as much as you'd hoped, then we suggest speaking to your GP who should be able to recommend further treatment. There are some useful resources and websites at the back of the book.

If you answered B–D then we're very chuffed for you and things can only get better from here if you keep putting what you've learned into practice.

2 **Which specific skills and strategies did you find particularly helpful?** Make sure you continue to incorporate them into your day-to-day life so they become second nature.

3 **Which of the 'takeaways' listed at the bottom of all the chapters particularly struck a chord?** Write them down on a notepad or in your diary so every time you need a pick-me-up you can flick through and motivate yourself.

4 **What support network do you have to help you maintain what you've learned?** Consider telling family and friends what you're doing if you haven't already. Their encouragement will be invaluable and motivational – and talking things through can give you some clarity or a different perspective. It might also show you the funny side of a situation. Laughing at yourself and the situation will immediately lift your mood and make you feel lighter, happier and more able to cope.

5 **What possible obstacles do you see in the future that might throw you off course?** Write them down and then work through any possible solutions.

6 **Consider whether or not you have really given this a chance.** If you have then that's brilliant. If you haven't, then ask yourself why. If you don't address your sleeping problems they'll keep returning. Being proactive about tackling them will make you feel so much better. You have nothing to lose by giving it a go.

7 **Do you now only use your bedroom for sleeping and sex?** If not then are you going to?

8 **Have you been putting your wind-down and relaxation routines into practice and if so, have they helped?** Are you going to continue using them even as your sleep improves? Even when things get better you shouldn't dismiss all of the positive changes you've made – glugging coffee at night and working until the small hours will only invite insomnia back into your life.

9 **Go through the tick list of symptoms in Chapter 2 again. Are there many changes for the better?**

10 **When are you going to start thinking differently about sleep?**

    A I already have   D Next week

    B Today   E Next year

    C Tomorrow   F I don't care

There are no right or wrong answers to these questions. This is a chance to assess how you feel now and if there are any specific areas you want to concentrate on. You now have the tools to improve your sleeping patterns – how you use them is up to you. A fundamental message of this book is realising that you have choices. If you're excited about making changes then we salute you. It's really hard, but very rewarding. And it works.

If there are some bits of the book that you haven't tackled yet, go back and try again, reminding yourself what you're meant to be doing and why. It's incredibly difficult to change your behaviour and the way you think, especially when habits will have been built up over many years. However, it is possible. Often just considering doing things differently is the hardest bit – and you're well past that stage now. Don't put undue pressure on yourself to change overnight: you're not likely to go from three to eight hours in a few weeks. These things take time, but it's time well spent. Make a date to re-read the book in a month, six months or a year's time to see how differently you feel then and to keep the ideas fresh in your mind. And keep flicking through your notebook. It'll be really motivating to see how far you've come and to remind yourself of the tips and tricks that helped before.

Now you're hopefully sleeping a bit better you can start planning for the future. We want you to make goals that you can take forward to give you a sense of direction. Pick something that you feel you could still work on – perhaps learning how to relax properly or how to manage stress. Plan to concentrate on the relevant strategies over the next month and update your sleep diary taking note of any new changes. In one month (make sure you specify a date in your diary so it's 'official') evaluate how you've got on and if you need to make any more changes. Remember: little adjustments add up to a big difference.

Change can be frightening, but everything in this book is designed to positively influence how you sleep and how you think and feel about sleep. That can only be a good thing! Good luck with everything and remember you're not alone and you *can* sleep well.

Further reading

Colin Espie, *Overcoming Insomnia and Sleep Problems* (London, Constable & Robinson, 2006)

Michael Perlis, Mark Aloia and Brett Kuhn, *Behavioural Treatments for Sleep Disorders* (London, Elsevier, 2011)

Dennis Greenberg and Christine Padesky, *Mind over Mood: A Cognitive Treatment Manual for Clients* (New York, Guilford Press, 1995)

Useful websites

MIND, The National Association for Mental Health: www.mind.org.uk

Time to Change: www.time-to-change.org.uk

The Sleep Council: www.sleepcouncil.org.uk

The Perfect Sleep Environment: www.perfectsleepenvironment.org.uk

The British Snoring and Sleep Apnoea Association: www.britishsnoring.co.uk

The British Sleep Society: www.sleepsociety.org.uk

Moodjuice – Sleep Problems: www.moodjuice.scot.nhs.uk/sleepproblems.asp

The Centre for Clinical Interventions: www.cci.health.wa.gov.au/resources

The Mental Health Foundation: www.mentalhealth.org.uk

The American Mental Health Foundation: americanmentalhealthfoundation.org

The Beck Institute: www.beckinstitute.org

Cruse Bereavement Care: www.cruse.org.uk

Relate: www.relate.org.uk/home/index.html

Frank: friendly confidential drugs advice: www.talktofrank.com

Alcohol Concern: www.alcoholconcern.org.uk

The British Psychological Society: www.bps.org.uk

The British Association for Behavioural & Cognitive Psychotherapy: www.babcp.com

Samaritans: www.samaritans.org

Acknowledgements

Thanks to all the people who believed in these books and helped to make them happen. Big thanks to our wonderful families, particularly Ben, Jack, Max and Edie. Also to our agent Jane Graham Maw for brilliant advice, our editor Kerry Enzor for her contagious enthusiasm and Peggy Sadler for her unsurpassed design skills. Jessamy would also like to thank the psychologists, health professionals and patients who have educated, supported and inspired her.